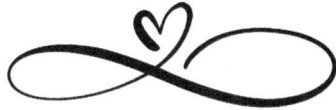

Praise for
The Power of a Conscious Athlete

Cindy's life's work has been the search for excellence and balance using sport as a vehicle to fully realize one's dreams. She has helped thousands of people to navigate their way through life's challenges and face roadblocks with her gentle hand and positive perspective. Never pushing, but guiding with approaches gleaned from a lifetime of study and a genuine passion for helping people. Whether you are an elite athlete looking for an edge or someone searching for a way to enrich your life, this book can help you.

–Sue Holloway
Canadian Sports Hall of Fame Olympian,
Cross Country Skiing and Sprint Kayak,
1979, 1980, Motivational Speaker

"It's about the journey, not the destination." Cindy embodies these words. Cindy's knowledge, approach, and presence have truly impacted my life. Cindy's depth is well beyond her coaching and training. The knowledge and insights Cindy has shared with me over the years are now captured in this book. Her coaching not only allowed me to complete five Ironman races (with the desire to do more), but more importantly, helped me understand the true meaning of, "it's about the journey, not the destination." On the surface, this book is about training for endurance sports, but if you read it carefully and reflect, you will find it is deeper than that.

—Growson Edwards
Serial Entrepreneur, Husband, Father, and Athlete

I have known Cindy my whole life as she is one of my mom's best friends and past coach. She is someone I lean on when my heart and soul need someone to talk things out with. Cindy leads with her whole heart and fills any room she walks into with love. This book is crucial for the athlete, but more importantly, for the human behind the athlete, to achieve deep success.

—Maddy Schmidt
Canadian Olympic Canoe-Sprint Kayak Team Member, 2020

For athletes interested in achieving peak performance, *The Power of a Conscious Athlete* is the book for you. Author Cindy Deugo focuses on setting intention and leveraging the mind and body harmoniously to achieve at the highest level one can imagine. As the coach of my son's high school crew team, I was able to witness Cindy Deugo teach each student athlete how to maximize their performance in a 100 percent positive atmosphere. She has the ability to translate to anyone how world-class athletes achieve greatness in sport. The tips, lessons, stories, and up-to-date sports science in this book are priceless. I highly recommend *The Power of a Conscious Athlete* to anyone who is interested in optimizing their performance in sport and in life.

—Jonathan Perrelli
Seven-Time Entrepreneur Turned Venture Capitalist

I met Cindy amongst the paddling community and we connected instantly. Both on and off the water, I've thoroughly enjoyed our conversations about career, sport, and the interactions with people in our lives. Cindy has a positive and supportive approach while challenging you to meet your goals with an open mind toward what is possible. This book shares a number of thoughtful concepts to explore with relevant examples that will resonate with so many. I felt encouraged to give myself the room to think and grow in new ways. Enjoy the read!

–Jane Labreche, PhD
Exercise Physiologist

I seek those who hold sacred the inner journey. For it is they who inspire me to search within, to free myself from the self-inflicted judgements that limit my growth, and at the same time, encourage me to open my heart with kindness towards myself. With all the gifts Cindy possesses—accomplished athlete, expert personal trainer and coach, yoga instructor, and meditation teacher—I believe her most remarkable gift is her ability to accept people for who they are, meet them in the sacred space of possibility, and inspire them to cultivate the strength, stamina, and conviction to reach their performance and life goals. I highly recommend her book for anyone seeking a conscious, holistic path for becoming their personal best.

–Dr. Suzanne Nixon, PhD
*Integrative Psychotherapist, Mindfulness Meditation
Teacher, Student, Colleague, Friend*

As a professional hockey skating coach for the past 30 years, my clients include Olympians, NHL players, and thousands of college and youth players. In 2008, long before hockey players were doing yoga, I hired Cindy Deugo to create and teach "Hockey Yoga" to AAA and NCAA skaters at a summer speed camp. The players finished the week inspired by Cindy to look inside themselves to harness the power of their minds to get the most from their bodies, and "Hockey Yoga" became a permanent, and enormously popular, part of our curriculum. She is an elite multi-sport athlete that has trained, conditioned, and taught athletes of all types and a wide range of abilities. She has amassed a vast understanding of human kinetics and mental motivation and has developed an exceedingly rare coaching skill set. She is a world class expert in sports performance coaching with the tools to target the specific needs of athletes in their individual sport and guide them to the peak of their physical and mental capabilities.

–Wendy Marco
Owner of ColdRush Hockey
and the Washington Capitals Skating Coach

Cindy Deugo and I met on the Rideau River by Mooney's Bay, Ottawa, and it was an instant connection. We were both passionate about paddling in sprint kayak and became dear, precious friends through all our hours on the water together. When she moved away, she continued to define her way in athletics and training, working with others to help them believe in their own journey to become better athletes, finding the essence of who they are and developing that mind-body connection, which is so very important in pursuing an athletic career. *The Power of a Conscious Athlete* awakens the power they have within to attain better performances than they ever thought possible! This book is one every athlete needs to read to have more effective accomplishments.

–Marjorie Homer-Dixon
Olympic Kayak Paddler, 1968 (Mexico),
1972 (Munich), 1985 (World Masters)

To be a member of Cindy's world is to experience the passion and dedication with which she engages and performs her role in the appreciation of coaching and training principles. With a practice that features a personal "hands-on" approach to each individual, group, or team activity, she has acquired a broadly based collection of successfully applied concepts. Those proven concepts support the development and preparation of subsequent performance plans.

The success of this process utilizing this data initiated the response that has resulted in the publication of her book. The book explores how individual performance parameters might be combined with conscious principles to achieve improved performance.

–Lowell Miller, PhD.
Chemical Engineer, US Department of Energy

I needed help but had been unsuccessful finding someone with the skills needed to support an aging, undisciplined 62-year-old with long-standing injuries from life's adventures. After hearing her name several times, I met Cindy by chance at an informal gathering. I consider it the luckiest day of my life. Cindy meets you (your mind, body, and spirit) where you are. You learn quickly that making excuses or talking yourself out of doing something doesn't work, because she has the skills, depth and breadth of knowledge and experience to adjust her guidance to help you keep going and meet your goals. Sometimes my goal is simply to relieve pain and stay mobile and I feel like I get the same consideration and commitment as a star athlete. Whether you can work with Cindy one-on-one, in a workshop, or through her book, you will be better off for it!

–Joan Schultz
World Bank Regional Manager Administration East Africa

The
Power of a
Conscious
Athlete

The Power of a Conscious Athlete

Open Your Mind and Heart
to Maximize Performance

CINDY DEUGO

PYP Publish Your Purpose

For permission requests, write to the publisher, addressed "Attention: Permissions Coordinator," at the address below.

Publish Your Purpose
141 Weston Street, #155
Hartford, CT, 06141

PYP **Publish** Your Purpose

The opinions expressed by the Author are not necessarily those held by Publish Your Purpose.

Ordering Information: Quantity sales and special discounts are available on quantity purchases by corporations, associations, and others. For details, contact the publisher at hello@publishyourpurpose.com.

Edited by: Gail Marlene Schwartz, Chloë Siennah
Cover design by: Cornelia Murariu
Photography by: Alimond Photography Studio
Typeset by: Medlar Publishing Solutions Pvt Ltd., India

Printed in the United States of America.

ISBN: 979-8-88797-062-2 (hardcover)
ISBN: 979-8-88797-063-9 (paperback)
ISBN: 979-8-88797-064-6 (ebook)

Library of Congress Control Number: 2023904431

First edition, August 2023.

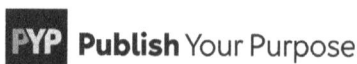

The information contained within this book is strictly for informational purposes. The material may include information, products, or services by third parties. As such, the Author and Publisher do not assume responsibility or liability for any third-party material or opinions. The publisher is not responsible for websites (or their content) that are not owned by the publisher. Readers are advised to do their own due diligence when it comes to making decisions.

Publish Your Purpose is a hybrid publisher of non-fiction books. Our mission is to elevate the voices often excluded from traditional publishing. We intentionally seek out authors and storytellers with diverse backgrounds, life experiences, and unique perspectives to publish books that will make an impact in the world. Do you have a book idea you would like us to consider publishing? Please visit PublishYourPurpose. com for more information.

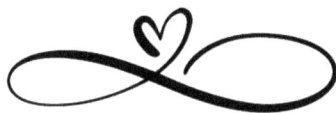

Dedication

To my family, who built the foundation of who I am.
To my children, Lily and Jaegar, the brightest lights,
most treasured gifts and unexpected teachers in my life.
To Dr. Lowell Miller who kept me on course,
graciously sharing his insights and years of experience.
To David Hazard who coached me from the "starting line"
of this book with patience and expertise.
To my training partners and friends who stood shoulder
to shoulder and encouraged me in my own awakening.

And to everyone along the way who saw in me
what I couldn't see in myself.

I am deeply grateful for you all.

Thank you.

The Power of A Conscious Athlete

To hold the balance and consider
the connection between mind, body
and spirit, we practice with joy,
with grit and deep determination.
Hold the breath and bone.
Hold the focus and pure presence.
Examine how the soul speaks
through this work in words
on the page, in years of worthy
attention, notes taken, all our
experiments meant to be shared.
We shape the future for each other
with our collections of tools
and the breakdown of our process.
Here is new illumination, here
is yet another way to know
how wonder gathers in us
just waiting to be expressed.
-j.suskin
2023

http://www.jacquelinesuskin.com/
Jacqueline Suskin is a poet and educator who has been teaching
workshops, writing books, hosting retreats and creating spontaneous
poetry around the world since 2009.

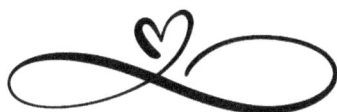

Contents

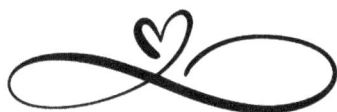

Foreword

O ver 35 years ago, I walked into the Rideau Canoe Club after moving to Ottawa, Canada. The first person I met there was Cindy Deugo, who welcomed me to their club with open arms. When I met Cindy, I was a kayak paddler who had dreams of representing Canada in my sport, but I was struggling to figure out how to get there. Cindy became a lifelong friend; first, as teammates at the Rideau Canoe Club, and later, as my coach guiding me to my full potential as an athlete. Today, I continue to benefit from the tools and confidence she gave me so many years ago—not only in sport, but in my career as a firefighter. I am proud to call her a friend and mentor.

As a young athlete, I was all about the hard work, putting in the kilometers on the water, always trying to do more. I was a training champion, but could not transfer my training to competition. When I began to work with Cindy as a coach, I was not as fast as I should have been, and felt let down by my own hard work. Under her guidance, I learned that it's not all about going out and hammering my body day after day. What works for some athletes was breaking me down and making me slower. After working with Cindy for a year, I went from a Provincial C-level athlete to a Canadian National Team member and proudly represented Canada at the 1987 Pan Am Games in Indianapolis, winning two silver medals.

Cindy has a keen ability to figure out what motivates her athletes and gets the very best out of them by treating them as an individual. She helps them figure out what drives them to perform and guides them into a deeper understanding of how they tick—or what she calls becoming a "conscious athlete." Cindy never applies a one-size-fits-all approach to coaching, which is why she is so successful. As an individual with unique skills and needs, she has learned how to look at the athlete as more than just a physical being who needs to train hard; she digs into the whole athlete and looks at the physical, mental, emotional, and spiritual strengths and challenges. Cindy knows when an athlete needs a push, and when they need to stand down; she teaches her athletes how to look inside and find the pieces that already exist within them, bring them out and help them shine, both as an athlete and human being. I still use many of the skills I learned under Cindy's guidance. I truly believe the confidence I gained as an athlete has transferred to my profession, where I have climbed the ranks to Deputy Chief, the first woman to achieve that rank in my department of 1,400 members.

This book is a goldmine for any athlete or coach working toward becoming not only better at their sport, but a stronger and more conscious person. It takes all the lessons Cindy has learned over her career as an athlete, coach, mentor, student, and academic, and teaches the reader how to look inside as a whole person, dig deep into their true purpose, and thrive in consciousness.

–Louise Hine-Schmidt
Deputy Chief, Ottawa Fire Services

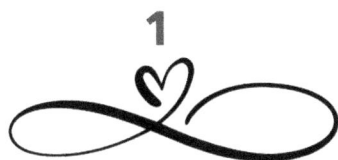

1

My Story

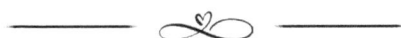

*How vain is it to sit down and write
when you have not stood up to live.*

—Thoreau

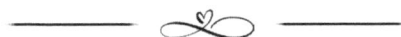

After many years of being unconscious myself, the slow road to consciousness along with my own wake-up calls, awakening, and insights led me to writing, or as I like to say, "birthing" this book. The best teachers are those who practice what they teach. Today, I am living a life much more in alignment with who I am. What I have to offer as a coach is grounded in an understanding of my athletes as human beings, not just as their goals and accomplishments. My education and certifications, along with over four decades of experience as an athlete, coach, trainer, instructor, therapist, and teacher have all taught me the lessons I am offering you in this book. Let me share with you where I began, my own unconsciousness, the price I paid along with the two-by-fours in the head, and the wandering off course I endured myself.

My Wake-Up Call

I found the sport of flatwater paddling in my late teens. Along with the success I had there, I found friendship, a sense of purpose; something that distinguished me from my previous persona of the overweight, unathletic girl. The Rideau Canoe Club in my hometown of Ottawa, Canada was a place where I felt like I belonged. I discovered that being an athlete could be rewarding in many ways, and I was hooked. That first summer of paddling in 1979, I lost 30 pounds, won gold medals at National-level competitions, traveled to new places, met Olympians, and made friendships that have endured over my lifetime. It didn't take long for my identity to wrap around this new found athlete. I started training in other sports and for the first time, considered myself a true athlete. I had found something that defined me in a positive way. The fitter I became, the better I felt. So I started demanding more from my body and added running and weight lifting to my daily routine.

Four years later, I was a 22-year-old university student diagnosed with the female athlete triad of tibia stress fractures, no menstrual cycle, and an eating disorder. I had unconsciously begun to deplete my body of energy reserves. Despite that early wake-up call from my maladaptive coping behaviors, I still tried to run on my broken shins. I didn't know what else to do or how to stop. I was unconscious of the fact that I had become my own worst enemy and was driven by the deeply buried voice of an "inner critic." No matter what I did, "good enough" was always just out of my reach. I added triathlon to my arsenal in 1983 and had great success in those early days of the sport. Still, the voice in my head reminded me that I was not worthy of the praise I received for any accomplishment.

I became a mother in my 30s and used multisport as a way to deal with living continents away from friends and family and to cope with an unhappy, unraveling marriage. I followed my husband at the time to Barbados, Florida, and then to Virginia. The woman I was had disappeared, literally and figuratively, to nine percent body fat just six months after my second child. I was fast, but I was a hollow and fragile shell of the person I wanted and pretended to be.

Outwardly, I received a lot of positive reinforcement for looking the way I did and for my achievements in sport. Winning races while raising two small children got me attention for being a "superwoman." My light, lean body was envied and complimented. That all reinforced the notion that I believed I had to be "perfect" in every way. I *must* have been doing great if everyone told me I was, right?

Sure, there were hints that not everything was in perfect balance and harmony. "But c'mon," I thought. "Whose life is perfect?" Who was I to complain about this uneasy feeling I had of living a life that was not the one I had signed up for? There was no happily ever after for anyone, was there?

In my late 30s and early 40s, I hunkered down for the long haul of being divorced and raising two children in an unfamiliar country. I took on the Ironman four times along with countless other triathlons, marathons, and road races to help dull the pain of a life I had not signed up for or ever imagined. I prided myself on being able to move mountains. In my mind, there was no such thing as an obstacle; I only had to push against it to get it out of my way. Yoga and meditation (which were just coming into vogue for athletes at that time) were, for me, practices in service of getting stronger, more fit, and—frankly—a way to bypass my chronic back pain and perform better in races. At first, yoga wasn't a way for me to develop a deeper awareness of myself and my motivations, but it didn't take long for it to start cracking me open.

Ironman also taught me lessons I will never forget.

My first was the Great Floridian in 1996. I wanted to support a friend that was racing. I had been racing for 13 years, done a Half Ironman in 1987, and figured, how hard would it be to double the distance? That day taught me how skilled I was at dealing with adversity. I "trained" with my friend for the six weeks after making that decision leading up to the race, and I found out what it was like to bite off more than I could chew. On the swim, I found myself thinking about the state of my unraveling marriage and ended up way off course. It was a strong parallel to how I felt in my life. Then, 70 miles into the bike portion of the race, I lost feeling in my left leg. I had put my own bike together after traveling and not marked how high my saddle should be. Guessing the height was not a good idea. My back gave out 90 miles into the 112 mile bike. The first three miles of the marathon were questionable as to whether I could limp my way through the next 23.2 miles. I realized in those long, arduous miles that my ability to cope, adapt, adjust, endure, and detach from outcomes—skills I had learned in my crazy childhood—were good skills to have. It wasn't pretty or fast, but that race was a strong invitation to wake up to not being defined by the outcome.

Ironman New Zealand in 2000 was a peak experience in my racing life. I used a spiritual skillset I had never tried before and had learned at Mark Allen and Brant Secunda's Sport and Spirit workshop back in 1999. Those skills included a deeper reminder of aerobic heart rate training, the power of mantras to get through difficult times on the course, how to stop fear and doubt in their tracks, and using the significance of prayer arrows and ceremony to tap into higher powers. I had never consciously called on something bigger than or so deep within myself to help me through a race or any other challenge in my life, and when I did, the results spoke for themselves: I had the best race of my life. There was no attachment to outcome. It was the beginning of being able to focus on something deep inside, a quieter voice that was different from the inner critic I had been unconsciously listening to for so long. It was the race that opened my own eyes and woke me up to limitless possibility and peak performance.

Four years later, Ironman Lake Placid reinforced my idea of what was possible, and I performed again beyond my wildest dreams. The course was perfect for me. The swim was in a crystal clear lake that had a cable you could simply follow to stay on course. The bike portion was a two-loop hilly course that required patience and strength, and it tapped into my capacity to deal with the familiar roller coaster of life. Running off the bike required having saved enough energy to run a marathon while being mentally prepared for its hills and the demands of being able to stay steady and strong. It was another race that reminded me of my ability to endure, but now, with a respectable time. I crossed the finish line with my two children hand in hand and knew that I could launch not only myself but also both of them into a future none of us could predict.

The next year, Ironman Canada, in contrast, held a mirror up to the thing I was most afraid of looking at: my own weaknesses. How could I reconcile a DNF (Did Not Finish) with the superwoman I thought people believed me to be? Who would listen to me, care for me, or love me when I stepped off the course of one of the biggest races of my life with 12.2 miles still to go? Those mountains I prided myself on moving, this time *literally* the Canadian Rocky Mountains, taught me a hard lesson. Sometimes you push your limits, and other times those limits push back. When sickness and overtraining forced me off the course, I had no frame of reference to tell me that it took a lot more strength to admit weakness and stop than it did to "be strong" and force myself to continue while brutalizing my body. That course pushed back and set a limit for me in a way I had never experienced before. Being vulnerable was not as scary in reality as it had been in my mind. People still loved me and respected me even though I had "failed." It was another lesson in my own waking up process, but it still took years of hard lessons to see that.

As I moved towards 50 and through menopause, I began to struggle with my health. I found myself feeling drained, sore, and unmotivated. My body was not cooperating like it used to. Some days I had the strength I had always counted on, and other days I felt like a weakling who had never lifted a weight in their life. I turned to an extra cup of coffee in the morning, ibuprofen along with my vitamins, and naps to recover from even a light workout. My heart rate told me I was not as fast as I used to be. My go-to strategy was always to push; to rest more was to give in to weakness, and I still couldn't possibly do that.

Something was wrong, that was undeniable, but instead of admitting I needed to rest, I opted to think I was sick. Maybe some antibiotics, an MRI, an explanation of my symptoms, and a solution from the medical community would get me back on track. They suggested it could be Lyme Disease or even MS, but no one in the medical community had concrete answers for me. If I wasn't "sick," what was going on in my broken and tired body?

My sister-in-law was the first to crack me open to the hard truth: I might need to rest. She used her Body Code and PSYCH-K energy worker skills to delve deep inside me and uncovered issues I had been wrestling with since my youth. Past issues and unconscious beliefs that had been buried were impacting me in ways I was unaware of. In my state of exhaustion, I no longer had the energy to deny that something deep inside me, operating outside of my awareness, was draining me of vitality and health. She shined the light on what I had kept in the dark. In that cracking open, I began to realize that changing my life could start with changing my beliefs. "There is no doubt that human beings have a great capacity for sticking to false beliefs with great passion and tenacity… I was exhilarated by the new realization that I could change the character of my life by changing my beliefs." (Lipton, 2008) Instead of being a victim of my reality and life, I discovered I could become the creator of it. And so the shift of consciousness began.

For so many years of my life, my unconscious and emotional body drove my physical body. False beliefs I had about myself—feelings of unworthiness, being undeserving of love—all drove me to try to prove I was worthy and deserving through success in sport. Being fit and strong was a good cover, but the fears remained under the surface. There was no changing those beliefs with any amount of physical success. The emotional misalignments pushed my physical body until it was drained and broken. I was unable or unwilling to look inside for years. I was like a junkie going after a fix to feel better, but as we all know, *nothing that goes on outside of us is going to fix what is going on inside of us.* It was easier to deal with physical pain than it was to deal with emotional pain. Sometimes there has to be ruin before transformation, a breakdown before a breakthrough.

Breaking down physically forced my emotional body to come into awareness. Change started from the inside out so my emotional body could come into alignment, old beliefs could be uprooted, and sport could be used to *serve* a healthy body rather than *push* an exhausted one. I understood that our perception and beliefs are what ultimately control our biology.

I have discovered that there are two ways to grow and to learn. The hard way is to be broken open, which is a long, slow, painful process, if there is anything left after the breaking. The other is to willingly shed that which no longer works—a much more conscious and painless way. We can either wait until it is too painful *not* to change or decide to make the changes as soon as we realize our old ways no longer serve us.

Eventually I found myself in the office of an acupuncturist, a doctor of Chinese medicine. He turned the mirror on me and forced me to look at what was really going on. He called my symptoms "the perfect storm." My energy meridians were completely out of balance. Hormones and the digestive system were the big culprits. Menopause had hit hard, and the energy I was putting into my body was not being processed properly. He told me it was like I had been using an "energy credit card," spending like I had an infinite supply. When the credit card bill came due, I had no energy in the bank to pay it with. My reserves were exhausted, and the only way to fill them back up was to make some changes that were long overdue and hard for me to swallow. Rest? Really? Look after myself better? Put myself first? Go for a walk instead of a run? Do yoga for the sake of self- and other-awareness, rather than to help me place higher in my age group? No more red wine or gluten? Tomatoes and peppers are now my enemy?!

Most of us never make a change until it is too painful not to change. That had long been one of my favorite sayings when I dealt with other people—those who I could see were looking for something in their life to change. After observing unhealthy patterns and habits, I would tell them through my own experience that *the only thing we can change is ourselves.* Until we realize what is at stake, see all we lose out on for ourselves, we won't be able to take the necessary steps to transform. Change happens when the fear of things staying the same becomes greater than the fear of changing, when the status quo becomes scarier than the transformation.

Waking up in the process of change will show you how to do what is most important in life, and that is to grow. Change that leads to growth builds a life of purpose and intention.

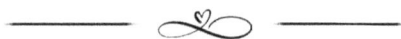

———— ✿ ————

You cannot control what happens to you, but you can control your attitude toward what happens to you, and in that, you will be mastering change rather than allowing it to master you.

—Sri Ram

———— ✿ ————

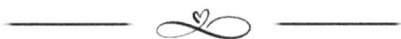

After decades of focusing on the outside, I was in serious need of a new set of inner life skills. The training that was supposed to be improving my health instead had unconsciously become a risk factor. The proof of that was etched into my cells, endocrine system, organs, and musculoskeletal system. I had, for years, been slowly and painfully broken open. With this health crisis, I was given the opportunity to finally choose to shed what was no longer working rather than be cracked open any further.

Overspending my energy had served me well until it no longer served me at all. The belief that if I *did* enough, I would *be* enough (because I believed I wasn't enough) was draining my vital energy.

There was no well to draw from, no reserve to tap into; it was time to start saving, time for me to make the necessary change.

Now I can look back with a clearer vision and a stronger understanding of the lessons I was being taught. I am still learning some of those lessons the hard way. The racing I do now is because I choose to, not because I have to or use it to fill a void or try to prove my worth. I even consciously stepped away from it for several years to learn the lessons from its absence. When I returned to racing, it was back to my roots as a paddler, and what a return it turned out to be when I finally listened to my heart, mind, and body.

I had the privilege of being invited to try out for the Canadian Women's Over 50 Dragonboat team to race at the World Championships in 2011. Dragonboat is an international sport that has its roots in China from 2,500 years ago. There are 20 paddlers, plus a steersperson and drummer. I had made the changes necessary for my body to heal and begun to practice the concepts I describe in this book. Not only did I make the team, but we won *four* gold medals and were undefeated at every distance we raced, from 200 to 2,000 meters. It was a peak experience in my life and a realization that there is more to sport than just working hard.

When you don't listen to the deep voice of your authentic self, it will only be a matter of time before it finds another way to demand your attention. As I tell all my athletes, the body *always* wins. Enduring physical pain rather than exploring emotional pain is certainly easier for a lot of us. It was easier for me until my body collapsed under me. When I finally had to listen to what those voices had been saying for so long, I had the opportunity to stop beating myself up and start standing in who I really am.

Standing in authenticity, I got to see what I was capable of, and I hope this book helps you to do the same. I extend an invitation to you into a higher level of consciousness. Use your sport as a vehicle not just to win awards or medals, but to find a deeper sense of purpose, a deeper sense of self, and into a life that brings you joy and peace.

...He then becomes the wise master, directing his energies with intelligence, and fashioning his thoughts to fruitful issues. Such is the conscious master, and man can only thus become by discovering within himself the laws of thought; which discovery is totally a matter of application, self-analysis, and experience.

—James Allen

An Invitation to Spirit through Sport

JOIN ME ON THE JOURNEY INWARD TO YOURSELF WHERE THERE IS NO FINISH LINE OR OUTCOME, SIMPLY THE OPPORTUNITY TO BE WHO YOU ARE AND TO FULFILL YOUR PURPOSE IN LIFE.

Sport is not an intermezzo, a meaningless interlude in our daily lives similar to play. Sport adorns life, amplifies it, and is to that extent a necessity both for the individual as a life function and for society by reason of the meaning it contains, its significance, its expressive value, its spiritual and social associations, in short, as a culture function.

—Sport Philosopher Klaus V. Meier

We have many skills as athletes that allow us to set goals, break barriers, challenge ourselves, and overcome adversity. We are strong, persistent, dedicated, fast, determined, visionary, and excited by our potential. In sport, we can *per*form to *trans*form. Performing is simply the execution of actions while transforming is to change in form, appearance, or structure. Sport opens in us the potential to become more than we can possibly imagine.

Physically, we are able. Beyond that, mentally and emotionally, we may have tapped into a deeper skill set that gives us a "better" outcome. Imagine what will be possible when we move to the untapped, uncharted spiritual level.

All spiritual cultures assert that we have a path to follow, a purpose, and that assertion involves several assumptions. It is most remarkable to me how we can realize those assumptions of ancient spiritual texts through sport, if only we bring awareness to the depths of our reasons to train and race.

One spiritual assumption is that **humans are called upon to develop and become better than they are.** Who of us, through sport, does not aspire to be better? We can learn to aspire not with better results, but with becoming a better human being.

Another assumption is that **to be most fully human requires individual choice and development by cooperative action with identifiable demanding conditions.** As long as we are conscious in our choice and development in the athletic realm, we quite necessarily must cooperate with the struggle and demands of our sport. When we participate in sport, we open ourselves up to vulnerability. We are exposed and at risk for criticism. We are at a very high level of engagement with ourselves and with our environment and at those heights we are invited to be fully present and human.

A third spiritual premise is that **there is something or someone outside and beyond us who is divinely interested as we succeed or fail in living up to our expectations.** Learning to be aware of some divine presence in our lives can be one of the most powerful foundations to stand on in whatever challenges we face, whether in sport, career, relationships, or even our health.

Finally, a fourth spiritual assumption is that **our stories/poems/ myths/codes reveal to us the elements of what it means to be human.** They allow us to move from one level of awareness in life to a higher one. That sharing gives us access to the "wisdom" of the culture. I hope that this book is one of those stories that shares what it is to be human through the vehicle of sport and brings a heightened awareness to the wisdom of our athletic culture. The path to wisdom and intelligence is to understand ourselves as human beings, not by theory or concepts but through direct experience. If we learn to pay attention, we can use athletic experience directly and profoundly in a meaningful way.

Consciousness is the next stage of our development and evolution. We are looking to understand this mind that inhabits us. The nature of consciousness is universal and primal and has long been known by ancient traditions and practices. There are cracks in the current science of understanding consciousness that are opening doors of possibility to the unexpected relationship between mind and matter interactions, between subjective consciousness and objective reality. (Glattfelder, 2019)

———— ∞ ————

In Tibetan, the word for "existence" is "sipa," which also means "possible." In existence, anything is possible, anything can happen.

—Ribur Rinpoche

———— ∞ ————

It will be the survival of the wisest and most conscious, not the fittest, on this planet. Wisdom makes us agents of change and transformation. To transform, we must change our essence, not our form;

we must transcend. And to change our essence, we must first become aware that a change is necessary. That awakening of consciousness is how you awaken your wisdom.

Consciousness will be a way for you to navigate this new course you are venturing out on. New skills and tools will be necessary, and you may have to give up things you already know and use. Your journey will be your own, and what you need, you already possess.

You simply need to look inside yourself to see that.

Looking inward is certainly not easy, but it is the only way to grow as an athlete and as a person. What you go through on the outside in training and competition brings out what is already inside of you. If you are not achieving the results you want, you are most likely more focused on what is happening *outside* of you rather than what is going on *inside* of you. I invite you to start down a new road to your sport, certainly one less explored and traveled, but one that you cannot deny when you decide to look inside yourself and discover the depths of your ability and your "self."

Awakening, becoming aware and conscious, requires a whole new skill set that will be unique to you. Some of those skills you already may possess, and even already be using, while others you will have to discover and practice. None of this is out of your reach if you are willing to turn your focus inward and trust who you are because of and despite your athletic training. We often won't make changes until it is too painful not to. We must come to realize that what used to serve us perhaps no longer does and start to look for new ways not only to train and compete, but also to act and behave in the whole, great expanse of our lives.

Through sport, we have the privilege if we so choose to find our life's purpose, not just our physical abilities. When you find out how far you can go and discover that once you arrive, there is no "there," you understand your limitations. Limitations are necessary because they give us something to try to go beyond. When you see your performance more as part of your journey than a definition of who you are, you have moved into the realm of consciousness and purpose. I am sure that most of you reading this book have put time, money, effort, perhaps your heart and soul into your sport. With that kind of commitment, it is certainly possible that we are looking to satisfy the human longing for fulfillment, for purpose, to make sense out of our lives. Perhaps sport can be looked at as your hero or heroine's journey, your call to adventure and to find meaning in your life. In finding meaning, you bring your gifts forth to share with others, and in the long run, become the hero or heroine you were meant to be.

I believe sport is a medium that allows us to express ourselves to our fullest potential and realize who we are really meant to be. Sport can reveal who we are if we move towards all our potentials: physical, emotional, cognitive, and spiritual. With an awakening consciousness, you may have already started to realize that your body is simply the vehicle of your soul. By reaching into the depths of who you are, you may be uncomfortable, but that is where all learning and growth takes place.

Becoming consciously aware, being present, awakening, looking inward, digging deep, and doing work harder than you are currently capable of accomplishing is what this book is really all about. It begins here and now: Wherever you are on your journey, doing this inner work will help you find whatever you are looking for in your quest for more from your sport and from your life. If you are participating in a sport or living a life void of self-examination, you are most likely not performing to your highest potential and living a less than authentic life. Making choices without awareness most often leads you down the road of unconsciousness, where you wake up one day wondering how the heck you got there, or wonder why the same things keep happening to you over and over again. On the other hand, if you are consciously choosing each day of your life with greater awareness of yourself, you can experience the best possible version of the athlete living inside you, waiting to emerge.

What You Will Learn

I want to teach you a skill set unlike any other you have focused on before. You will learn to examine your choices, your life, and answer some hard questions you may not have considered before. You will look at the cost/benefit ratio of the energy you expend in your sport and other areas of your life to make sure you are filling rather than draining your body, mind, heart, and soul. You can live a simple and deliberate life and consciously choose what you allow into your being. You will learn to move your body while restoring your vitality and perhaps broadening your awareness to the bigger picture. You will know what your big rocks are and learn to put them in your jar first.

Think of this book as your guide to developing a more acute awareness of your thoughts, feelings, actions, movements, and the choices you make. You will also find a voice that will lead you to a better athletic performance defined by something other than outcome, and perhaps even a better life defined by the new conscious athlete in you. You can start to observe your patterns of behavior, thought, and emotion just like you observe your patterns of movement. You will discover if those patterns are still serving you in ways that are consistent with your goals in your sport and aligned with you and the life you are living, or if you need to change them.

There are benefits to trying out the methods discussed in this book. In trying a new approach, you may find enjoyment rather than addiction, fulfillment rather than depletion, building relationships rather than breaking them down. Your body may be strong rather than fragile, and you may develop an attitude of flexibility, both mentally and physically, that allows you to find your way around the obstacles and limitations in your life and in your performance. Why flexibility? Because if you hold onto your current rigid mindset and body, you will not understand how sometimes you have to go backwards to go forwards, slow down in order to speed up, to listen and learn rather than think you know, and to be still rather than move. When you turn your awareness from outside of you to inside of you, the depths of you become accessible and powerful. Who you really are and what you are capable of can come to the surface as you take steps towards a more conscious and deliberate self.

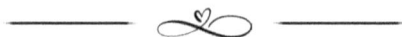

———————— ∿ ————————

When I let go of who I am, I become what I might be.

—Lao Tzu

———————— ∿ ————————

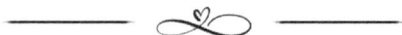

It takes courage to step outside the box, to forge new frontiers, to speak a different language about sport and performance. Some of you will not be ready to embrace some of the concepts in this book. Some of you may already be nodding knowingly at my message. Still others may have already figured this out and are ahead of me on this path of consciousness. I am passionate and excited about what is possible, about breaking barriers in ourselves and in our sport. As we all know, those barriers get broken all the time with new training methods, new technology, and new techniques. I hope to add to that long list of new ways by adding consciousness of ourselves. Perhaps the definition of what a successful athlete looks like will change. If you are connected to your inner being, the work you do in the outside world will have more quality. The outgrowth of your inner essence is your gift to those around you and to your outer world.

2

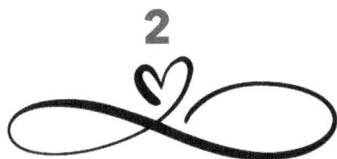

The Unconscious Athlete

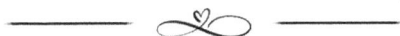

I have no doubt whatsoever that most people live,
whether physically, intellectually, or morally, in
a very restricted circle of their potential being.
They make use of a very small portion of their
possible consciousness…much like a man who, out
of his whole-body organism, should get into the
habit of using and moving only his little finger…
We all have reservoirs of life to draw upon,
of which we do not dream.

—William James

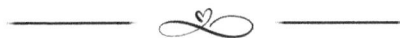

Anything is possible.

Impossible becomes *I'm possible* if you just add an apostrophe and a space.

If you have the desire to reach outside your comfort zone, to learn new skills, to grow beyond your wildest dreams, there is really only one thing you will have to do… and that is simply do something different.

This book will offer you something different. Something you may not have thought of before. Something that makes what you perceive to be impossible, possible.

And that is simply to become conscious.

A fundamental principle of quantum physics is that consciousness is responsible for the character of our lives. We are the creators of our life experiences. The origin of the modern concept of consciousness is often attributed to John Locke's Essay, "Concerning Human Understanding." He defined consciousness as the perception of what passes in a man's own mind (Locke, 1690). In 1903, the British philosopher James Allen wrote *As a Man Thinketh*, a book that tells us, "as a man thinketh in his heart, so he is." (Allen, 1903) We are literally what we think, and I would add what we feel, in our minds and in our hearts—with character being the sum of all our thoughts and feelings.

Consciousness is our awareness of what is, of what passes through our minds and our hearts. It is more than intellectually knowing; it is a deep inner knowing. Coming into consciousness allows you to move away from your fear and into your power and authenticity. Consciousness is a higher state of alertness and awareness that allows for habitual and limiting patterns of thoughts to become creative and original—and that is where possibility resides.

Change the Mind: Change the Film

If you change the way you look at things, the things you look at change.

—Wayne Dyer

The mind, and the ability to change it, is the next frontier of performance enhancement. One of my mantras is lose your mind to find your heart. We often consider losing our mind to be going insane, but consider if you will that, in losing your mind, you will go sane. If your mind is your brain in action or information being moved by your nervous system, then when you change your brain and that information (your thoughts), you change your mind. In changing your mind, you change your reality. You may think that changing your mind is hard to do or even a miracle. The book *A Course in Miracles* defines a miracle as simply a change in perception; that miracles arise out of a mind that is ready for them, and miracles are thoughts. (Foundation For Inner Peace, 1996).

Changing your thoughts changes your life and changes your world. The world you believe or the person you believe yourself to be may simply be what someone else told you about *their* perception of you. In shifting *your* perception, you have the opportunity to become who you choose to be and reach the potential you may not have been able to achieve with that change in your mind. Miracles cannot rest in an empty place. We need consciousness and certainty

> Changing our minds, our thoughts, and our beliefs just might be the most significant and powerful change of all.

for them to manifest. Certainty is the power that draws miracles into our lives. You can consciously shift your perceptions and in doing so, change your world.

The truth is that we create our own reality with the thoughts we think. Consciousness is still being explored in the scientific realm. There is no way to measure it or define it. It is a subjective term that sets up a paradox in that we know it is there, but don't quite understand what it is. We can't ignore that it is there. Peter Russell, a British author, physicist, and meditation teacher focusing on consciousness and spirituality, defines consciousness as a fundamental quality of the cosmos like space, time, and matter. He tells us, "Within our heads lies one of the most complex systems known in the universe" and "Our experience of the world is a representation of reality created by the brain." (Russell, 2014) The word consciousness in Buddhism was translated from the Sanskrit word *vijnana*, and refers to one's consciousness, self-awareness, or knowing; I am aware that I am aware. They believe the self and consciousness is a constantly changing stream of mental experiences. Russell and the Buddhists help us understand the connection between consciousness, our minds, and our reality with the image of a projector, along with our ability to change that reality consciously.

Let me explain.

There is a white light in the projector that passes through the film and is projected as an image onto a screen. When we are in a movie the-

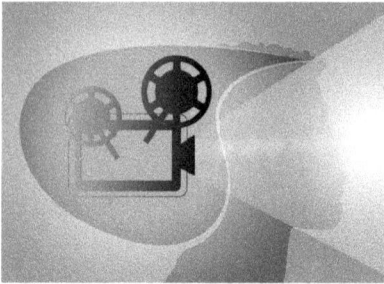

ater, our attention is on the story on the screen in front of us and we react to it almost as if it were real life. In reality, though, the images we are seeing are merely sculpted light that has passed through a filter. Metaphorically, the white light is our consciousness or our ability to experience; the film is our brain and our mind including our perceptions, intuition, thoughts, beliefs, feelings, memories. Our life, our reality then, is how our film—our mind—has sculpted our experience into our lives. Consider that we can change our lives, our selves, and our realities by turning and looking at the light (becoming conscious) instead of at the screen or making adjustments to the film we are putting that experience through. Unfiltered, that light, that consciousness, has the potential to become anything.

We usually don't make a change until it is too painful not to.

Changing our minds, our thoughts, and our beliefs just might be the most significant and powerful change of all.

We are caught in the paradigm of our existing understanding of our lives. To shift that paradigm takes courage, time, and patience, and may entail enduring ridicule and opposition from others and yourself. Eventually, that shift will be self-evident. Don't forget, we used to believe that the world was flat. It took Copernicus in 1543 to Newton in 1687 for that shift in belief to happen—144 years. Your thoughts and your mind are most likely even more resistant than that to shift.

Like any other skill you want to learn, from riding a bike to learning a new language, there are techniques to help you. Some will make more sense to you than others, but you will find your own set of tools to use for yourself. Your success in changing any interfering behavior or thought pattern depends on you being conscious of you. You need a conscious way of observing yourself and your life, a conscious method of regularly imparting life-energizing thoughts into your mind as often as possible. You need a way of thinking that consciously embraces what is good for your mind and body, your relational health, financial independence, self-actualization, and other essential aspects of your life.

Learning to program your mind and your thoughts along with your emotions for success is underestimated and overlooked, in my experience, until you step up to elite levels of training. How many of you reading this book practice thoughts like, *I love to compete* or *I love the energy of being in a field of fellow athletes and choose to focus on remaining present and in the flow*. Positivity, mental and emotional, can become an immense power in your life and in your sport if you practice it like any other skill where it is important for you to excel. There is only so far your body alone can take you. At World and Olympic level sport, most bodies have been honed to excellence. What separates the field is their mind and heart set.

One of the most positive athletes I have seen in the multi-sport world is Natascha Badmann. A six-time Ironman Hawaii winner, Natascha has had her share of battles out on the course at Kona. And she loves it. She's famous for her smiles and joy during the race, her positive attitude despite adversity, and inspiring many athletes around the globe. Her positive mindset and outlook are tools that she has sharpened to the point that they only help her in any situation. Her physical and mental strength is impressive when it comes to turning struggle into growth and generating positive energy from it.

> When was the last time you thought anything was possible? That your life was a blank canvas in front of you waiting for you to fill? That you were open to exploring more possibilities than you had yet imagined? When was the last time you challenged yourself, risked failure, and bit off more than you thought you could chew? When was the last time you accomplished something beyond what you thought possible, as you stepped up to the starting line of a race or the start of a game, unsure that you could even get to the finish line, but dared to try anyway?

Do you really understand what motivated you to enter your first game or race or why you continue to compete now? There is something about engaging in competition, not only in relation to others, but in relation to a power deep within ourselves, that can either hold us back or empower and change us. When you are aware of the motivating forces from within, you can use them to enhance your life rather than diminish it. If you unconsciously use sport as a way to cope with feelings of fear and unworthiness, you will most likely never find that sense of joy and worthiness, no matter how well you perform. You cannot tap into your real power if the motivation is coming from a place of fear and self-doubt.

Closing the Gap

In my 45+ years of experience as a professional trainer, coach, and athlete, I have not known anyone who has stepped up to their first starting line or tee, race, or game, without feeling vulnerable, fearful, or doubtful that they could finish it or win. I know many who crossed the finish line or played their game and felt the satisfaction, the sense of accomplishment, the deep knowing by the act of competing and pushing themselves to the limit and beyond. They knew they had somehow transformed themselves and perhaps even altered the course of their lives. Their blank canvas of possibility became etched with the word *athlete*. There was a weaving of new threads into the fabric of their life and a deeper knowing that what we learn in the moments of accomplishment and hours of training for those moments can radically change us and our lives, our relationships, our work, and our physical bodies.

Even more importantly, this deeper knowing can expand our minds and our spirits.

Sport can be used as a vehicle to an enhanced life or as a vehicle to cope with an existing one. The power to decide, regardless of what has been done up to this point, is in your hands.

This book will help you connect with that power—your own deeper level of consciousness—in ways that can transform you, as both an athlete and a human being. To do this, you must narrow the gap between consciousness and unconsciousness, that of which we are aware and that of which we are not. By narrowing this gap, you create more possibility and personal power than most people can imagine.

To begin exploring that gap, let me ask you some questions that you may not have answers for right now; just consider them as you discover how to move into consciousness. I suggest you take out a journal and write down your answers before you dive into the rest of the book.

- Do you train and race with complete awareness of what each and every workout is doing for you and why you are doing it? Are you driven by purpose or by addiction?
- Are you interested in performing better in your races, your relationships, and your life? Are you ready to live up to your potential?
- Would you like to learn how to tap into something that already exists inside you that you may not have even noticed was

there, something that can radically change the outcome of your training and your life?

- Are you willing to take a deep look inside yourself, to find out who you really are and what motivates you?

Most of us have been taught to train physically harder to get better, faster, fitter. There is another way to train. All you have to do is be brave, open, and conscious enough to look deep inside yourself and be willing to take control of what you think and how you feel.

If you are, I invite you to explore a new kind of awareness and a new way of being. I invite you to not just rely on what you have already done or learned, but to open up new territory and possibility.

"It always seems impossible until it's done."

—Nelson Mandela

A New Field of Competition

The skills you will encounter in this book are not for the faint of heart. They require a commitment to excellence beyond our bodies and performance, a willingness to challenge belief systems, and the courage to change ourselves from the inside out. Fear not, you are far braver than you realize and have already taken the first step in moving towards consciousness by picking up this book.

Every sport draws a diverse group to its starting line, arena, field, or court. Many of us who participate in those sports share common characteristics and a similar mindset. You may have started competing for one reason, stayed for a completely different one, and now wonder what more there is to learn from your career as an athlete. Some athletes have found freedom with their training, while others have unconsciously become captive.

What we are unconscious of may have just as much power (or perhaps even more) as the cognitive processes of which we are conscious. Our sport, identity, relationships, and even health can become compromised in that unconscious captivity. Is it possible that you are a hostage to your own unconsciousness? Are you open to deeply exploring what drives you as an athlete? See if you recognize yourself in any of the athletes whose stories follow. In these examples, I will illustrate what unconsciousness can look like and how it has the power to hold athletes captive.

CASE STUDIES

DAVE - AVOIDANCE

Dave had completed seven Ironman triathlons in four years. During that time, he had two young children with his first wife, he separated from and divorced her, and started dating a woman in his triathlon club. His daily routine on top of his 50-hour work week included early morning swims, midday runs, and evening bikes. Weekends alternated between bike/run workouts and children. There was not much room for anything else.

SUSIE - IDENTITY THEFT

Susie underwent knee surgery after repeated injuries she sustained over 10 years of playing soccer. She had tried new shoes, taping, icing, acupuncture, ART, massage, rest, and yoga, but nothing helped. Injury seemed to be the only thing on her mind and the only thing she talked about. Her whole identity and much of her conversation was wrapped around her knees and how they held her back.

GARY – EXCUSES

Gary was never happy with his hockey games. There was always a reason he didn't score more goals: He hadn't slept well the night before. His wingmen were not passing well. His defensemen were not doing their job. The ice surface was slow. He would have, should have, could have scored more goals. Frustrated in each game, he struggled against all the factors he could not control.

JULIA – NOT ENOUGH

Julia rarely said a kind word about herself. She diminished her body by pointing out her "jiggly thighs" while ignoring her beautiful running stride and smile. Most of her friends would have loved to have the body that she complained so much about. She weighed herself daily and that set her up for a day of focusing on whether she was "fat" or not. She was never happy with the times she posted race days and was sure that if she could lose weight, not only would she be happy, she would be fast.

CHARLIE – LOSING PASSION

Charlie had been racing for 25 years. He came into triathlon in the early days when we really didn't know what we were doing but did it anyway. He had always laughed at the mistakes he made on race day (like when he accidentally took the guy's shoes who was racked beside him in transition instead of his own and didn't even notice) and looked forward to getting up early each morning to train. But recently, it was harder for him to get out of bed. He had less joy on the bike, with increased intolerance of cyclists on the road. He enjoyed the people he raced and trained with, but he had lost his zest for racing and didn't find joy in logging yardage in the pool or miles on the run. He looked forward to emails about social events more than about group rides.

DEBBIE - COMPARISON IS THE THIEF OF JOY

Debbie went to 10K races to see who she could beat. It was never about enjoying her day—it was about her fellow age-groupers and whom she was there to compete against. She took more pleasure in beating people than in her own time, and she made sure everyone knew who she had conquered. It gave her some meaning or worth to "hang scalps" on her wall of those she measured herself against. Being better on the race course, regardless of the unrest in the other areas of her life, proved her worth. She was unfulfilled in her job, had no strong relationships left in her life outside of her sport, and never had the children she thought she would raise.

JACK - IDENTITY CRISIS

Jack had two sets of clothes: the suit he wore to work and the sweats he worked out in. Like Superman, he had two identities. He had to be at work or working out, and even when he was at work, he liked to make sure his Superman was somewhere noticeable, like the CrossFit gym sticker he placed on his day planner.

JOHN - OWN WORST ENEMY

John was an exceptionally skilled golfer. He had been playing since he was four years old. Now, at 40, he had a long career in the sport behind him that was never quite what he thought it would be. He had high expectations of himself when he played, and if his performance was not up to those expectations, he would swear, throw his clubs, and find someone or something to blame. He was never able to have a score that reflected the physical ability and skill level he had. Considering his mental and emotional game was not an option. Spending more time and money on his swing was what he believed would change his game.

I want to point out a couple of important factors about these stories of athletes and unconsciousness.

Each of these people got into the sport for a reason: identity, purpose, health, friendships, and maybe even a reason to get up early most days. When competing, they felt excitement and passion and a feeling of fulfillment.

In various ways, however, each has become hostage to a different need which has taken over. Let's call it a constant need to feed their egos, their emptiness, their boredom, their fear, and, in some cases, a reason to be. We are generally unconscious of these negative motivators and therefore risk the consequences of having them driving our actions.

All of these athletes have also lost power in some aspect of their lives, whether in relation to their motivation, their physical or mental state, or their emotional or relational well-being. This adds up to poorer overall performance, not only in athleticism, but in life.

Do consequences like that matter to you?

If they do, this book can help you.

Looking Deeper

Many of us look for something to get involved in, for great reasons at first, only to end up paying a price we never could have conceived of for our choice. Or we lose our way because we don't recognize the true power of an activity in which we found excitement and purpose at the outset.

Perhaps you recognized similarities in one of the examples above where you lost sight of your initial investment, got persuaded into a longer race, looked to be on a better team, took the credit for how many goals you got rather than acknowledging who assisted you, pushed friendships aside when they could no longer keep up with your skill level, or even convinced yourself that the status you got from your athletic achievements was more important than how you treat people. Maybe you haven't figured it all out yet, but you do know that there is something missing or something you have lost.

This book will help you find your way to a deeper awareness of how you got to where you are, guide you to where you want to go, and align your life consciously.

Imagine yourself out on a dark race course. You are moving forward, trying to navigate to the finish line. Without light, you are likely to run into some obstacles standing in your way that you just can't see. If you're on a field or in an arena that's unlit, it will be difficult to score a goal. If you're on a balance beam in a softly-lit gym, chances are you will lose your footing and fall. Turning up the light gives you a clear vision of what is in front of you and helps guide you to where it is you want to go without fear or consequence. We perform optimally, powerfully, and more confidently in the light.

Think of that light as consciousness or awareness illuminating your way out of the darkness of unconsciousness onto a clearer path of journeying towards your destination. You may even see things along the way you never noticed before and wonder how you missed them. That light—that consciousness—allows you to examine your life and yourself, your outer and inner world, with better tools and to develop a deeper understanding of what inspires and motivates you. Shining a light on yourself, your thoughts, your emotions, and your behavior can bring you to new heights in athleticism and in all other aspects of your life.

Unseen Forces

What if I told you there are some forces pushing you down a path, forces that currently lie beyond your control and are hidden from your awareness? When you find yourself not being able to relax unless you have worked out, or you choose to practice over going to a friend's barbeque, you may want to consider what is driving your choices. You may be completely unaware that there is a truth lying deep inside you, one you don't want to face. Maybe you are chasing something that always seems just out of your reach, like a carrot at the end of the stick. Perhaps you are haunted by a belief system imposed on you years ago.

If you recognize yourself in the athletes described above, you're in great company. Every one of us can benefit from gaining new insight about who we are and learn a new set of practices with which to develop ourselves. None of the examples are stories of "right and wrong," nor are they judgments about who these people are or the choices they make. They are merely observations of common themes and people that encouraged me to write this book to help athletes craft a more conscious, aligned, and purposeful life. Think of what you're being offered here as training for your inner being. Your inner being is your deeper, conscious, higher self that could also be called the essence of you or your soul. You've invested a lot in your physical or outer person. What if, by learning a new set of inner life skills, you could:

- Become better in your sport than you thought possible and, at the same time, more aligned/balanced with the other aspects of your life that may be missing or have been neglected?
- Move out of the stagnated, unconscious person you have become into being someone more authentic?
- Make more sense out of your life?

Through this book, you can develop a conscious awareness of who you are, where you are headed, and why.

You're probably thinking, "How? Let's get to that, please."

Hold on.

In the course of this book, you will explore the steps to consciousness, learn new skills and tools to deliberately enhance performance, develop a better understanding of yourself, and dig into your depths.

You will discover how to intentionally change and manage your thoughts, emotions, and beliefs to help you make powerful choices, come into alignment with your authentic self, and perform to your fullest potential. The benefits include enhanced performance, more fun, better health, along with a better understanding of why you choose to spend your precious time and energy in your sport.

Before we move into the important new skills you'll need to reach new heights of achievement and living, it's important to take a look at where you are right now. Why? Because most of us only invest ourselves in growth and change when the cost of staying the same is too high, or when we finally wake up to the fact that there is a way to change and to become greater than we currently are.

Where are you in this "awakening" process? Have you considered that you are creating your own reality or is this all something you have never thought about?

It will most likely be uncomfortable for you to awaken. It's important for you to know that this discomfort will be unfamiliar and your brain is wired to move away from it. Trust me. I have spent years in the familiar discomfort of unconsciousness, taking baby steps down the unfamiliar road of consciousness. If you consider waking up a process rather than an event, an opportunity to learn rather than to think you know it all already, a practice rather than a game or competition, you will most certainly find yourself not only awakening into a higher state of consciousness, but also more comfortable operating in this new state of being.

> Where are you in this "awakening" process? Have you considered that you are creating your own reality or is this all something you have never thought about?

"The duration of an athletic contest is relatively short, while the training for it may take many weeks of arduous work and continuous exercise of self-effort. The real value of sport is not the actual game played in the limelight of applause but the hours of dogged determination and self-discipline carried out alone, imposed and supervised by an exacting conscience. The applause soon dies away, the prize is left behind, but the character you build is yours forever."

—Unknown

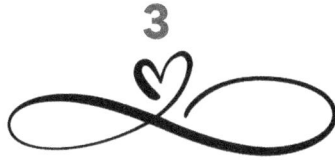

3

The Wake-up Call

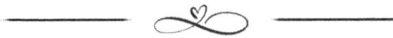

There is no coming into consciousness without pain.

—Carl Jung

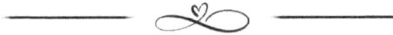

Waking Up

There are many ways we wake up to the relationship between performance and a new level of consciousness.

Some of us listen to the quiet whispers from within, gently summoning us to find new ways to live our lives. If we are sensitive and pay attention, we will only need the light touch of a feather. If we resist learning, however, we'll need a sledgehammer to learn the same lesson. Sometimes we wander off course and find our way back quickly; sometimes we wander for long periods of time without ever realizing it. Maybe it is in the wandering that we learn the most about ourselves. As the saying goes, "Not all who wander are lost."

Whether we wake up slowly or quickly, a new light will dawn. Whether you have wandered way off course or just a few steps, that light can guide you back on course. The light is telling us, "You have the chance to figure out who you really are and why you're doing what you're doing. Let that self-knowledge act like a beacon."

One of the most competitive athletes I coached, Derek, was racing in a sprint-distance triathlon and found himself in a group of elite cyclists out on the bike course ahead of the rest of the field. The race was grassroots and did not have a strong volunteer base, so the turns on the bike were not as apparent as they could have been with better race marshaling. At one point, the group missed a turn and ended up off course. Derek had raced the course before and had a subtle sense early on that they were lost. Given the competitiveness of the pack, however, he thought, "Maybe the course is different this year, or maybe I've forgotten the turns." Something inside him was telling him he was going off course, but he didn't trust his gut. He was caught up in the competitiveness of the pack. Once the whole group realized there had been no course markers for longer than expected, a sense of panic flooded in and they tried to retrace their steps. By that point, they had all lost out on placing in their respective age groups. Eventually, they found their way back on track, completed the bike, and ran harder than they thought possible to try to regain the time they had lost.

If you have ever had the experience of being off course, you know the panic you feel when you realize it. You work as hard as you can to get back on course, pressing as best you can to make up for the time you feel you've lost.

Be Here, Now.

Athleticism demands that we be as fully present as possible. There is a presence in competition that demands you to be in the "now." The intensity brings heightened awareness. We don't live in that intensity in regular life. More often than not, our mental and emotional states keep us locked in the past or toss us far ahead of where we are now, into the future. When this is so, we are impaired when it comes to recognizing that we are off course. Unless we develop our own "course marshal" to direct us—a clear, fully-present sense of awareness—we may not get back on course, and we are left wondering how and why, after such a great start, we wandered.

Here's the thing: Your sporting life exists in the greater context of your *whole life*. You can't compartmentalize it and say, "My regular life is *over there*, outside and apart from what I do as an athlete. What happens while I'm competing is *separate* from what is going on in the rest of my life." There is no real wall within us that divides our life from our athleticism.

So many influences from our life at large can pull us off course when we compete—and, unfortunately, we can remain unaware of them until they harm us or our performance. Staying in the darkness of unawareness can destroy your body and your life.

Look at the athletes who diminish themselves no matter how well they perform. It's never good enough, and they are never good enough. Do you know anyone like Sara, who is never happy with her race results? No matter how fast she runs a 10K, she beats herself up for not running faster.

How many of us know the athletes who try to cope with some crisis in their lives by numbing themselves with competition and training? For example, Steve, whose world unraveled when his son was arrested for drugs. Instead of spending more time at home, he spent more time on his bike trying to cope with the fallout in his family.

We can all translate the lesson of the lost cyclists into our own experience. We get off course in our training, in our performance, and in our lives because we become misled by a faulty sense of direction or an unwillingness to trust what our gut—or what our entire body—is trying to tell us. If we develop a strong sense of not only our goals, but of the signals we are getting from within ourselves, then we will be able to get back on course quickly, ensuring we will find our way not only to our training, fitness, and competitive goals, but also to our most authentic selves and lives.

Too often, though, we resist or ignore signals because of being unconscious. Our inner GPS can be turned off or dulled, so we don't even pick up the signals that we are headed in the wrong direction. The truth is, we need to pay attention to and pick up every signal we can because it can be telling us something important. The more you ignore your inner GPS, the louder it will have to speak to you. Learning to listen to the whispers and intuition of your body earlier rather than to the yelling of it later will most certainly help you reduce the consequences of having not paid attention.

Sports and life don't exist apart from each other. The way we are in life is the way we will be on the field of competition and vice versa. Developing a total and deep sense of awareness can keep us on course toward the best life possible. And isn't that, really, a hugely important goal? Learning to step onto the playing field of consciousness will help you on the playing fields of your sport and your life.

As you explore physical barriers, for example, you will find limitations that challenge you and encourage you, or perhaps even force you, to seek other ways to achieve your goals. Or perhaps those barriers will help you look at success in a whole new light. In sport and in life, you cannot change what you are not aware of or what you don't notice. Conscious awareness can begin to grow and help you in more ways than you may currently be able to imagine, supporting you in using your time and energy wisely. Noticing behaviors that no longer serve you will help you make the necessary changes to stop them.

We all know the stories of NFL players who may lead the league in yards rushing but drive their cars at dangerous speeds or abuse their wives and girlfriends. The cyclists who use performance enhancing drugs to win medals but deny it. The athletes who, despite their phenomenal achievements in sport, still suffer from depression.

If you want to live a life that is full and fulfilling, you must develop a sense of who you are, why you do what you do, how your thoughts (what passes through your mind) and how you feel (what passes through your heart) encourage, define, and represent you. Shine a light on your dark; your unknown, unexplored potential, and on what holds you back. Then shine that new light of awareness out into the world you want to live in.

Developing Awareness: Coaching to Consciousness

Athletes contact me to coach them for races of all distances and for sports of all kinds. Some are stepping up to their first sprint triathlon, and others are trying to become first string players. Most of them are starting from some awareness that they need help, direction, or guidance in their training. They all want to work as hard as they possibly can in order to achieve their goals. They want some "method to their madness," so to speak, some carefully crafted, well thought out, and individualized plan to navigate their way not just to the finish line but also to the starting line.

My vision as a coach has always been to be a midwife to the human spirit. I see qualities and strengths inside my athletes that they may not see in themselves, and I encourage them to give birth to those qualities and strengths through the vehicle of sport. When they understand why they choose to do the things they do with regards to their sport and their lives, their level of consciousness increases, and they move in the direction of purpose rather than aimlessly wandering off course. If they only want to get to a finish line as fast as they possibly can, or rack up as many wins as possible, I am not the coach for them. If their motivation is to learn something about themselves, explore who they are, grow as a human being, show up better in all areas of their lives in that journey to the starting and finish line, then I am happy to provide whatever assistance I can.

It is important to me to work with the whole person, not just the athlete. To help athletes be in alignment and balance in all aspects of their lives is what I aspire to do as a coach. The interconnectedness of our lives and our sport is undeniable. Our performance cannot help but improve when the other areas of our lives support and balance our athletic life.

One person that stands out as an athlete I felt in alignment with was Greg. He contacted me to coach him early one spring after doing two local sprint distance events the previous race season with unexpected success. He had won his age group in both races. He had two young children, was recently divorced, and had lost 75 pounds in the past two years. I had him fill out my initial athlete questionnaire to get a feel for who he was, what his goals and history were, and what he was looking for in a coach.

I read over his answers on the questionnaire and decided that I might be interested in working with him. We met at a local coffee shop to see if our personalities and philosophies were consistent enough to make a good team.

He showed great awareness of his strengths and weaknesses. He ranked himself highest for motivation, commitment, and positive attitude, and lowest for flexibility. He had a tight neck that flared up after too many hours at a computer and a tight IT band that talked to him when he didn't take the time to stretch. Now that he was single and had his children on a schedule he could work around, he had more time to train. The good news, to me, was there was no compromising the time with his children; he was unavailable to train when it was his evening or weekend. He held his children higher in priority than his training. There are training plans and coaches that push people, that require an over-focus on and sacrifice for their sport that can lead to imbalances in other areas of their lives. If Greg felt at all guilty or torn while training for his Ironman and taking time away from his children, his performance could not help but be compromised. As his coach, it was my job to keep him in alignment and in a positive state of emotion.

He was relatively new to swimming and wanted technical help, was confident on his bike, and could already hold a 6:30 pace for a 5K. His goals for the upcoming race season included being highly competitive in his age group at the shorter Sprint and Olympic distances and competing in a full Ironman with a time of less than 13 hours. He also wanted to have a body mass index in the single digits. Eventually, he wanted to do multiple Ironman-distance races and be an inspiration and example to his children and family. His weekly training had developed into a doable routine that he wanted to build focus and goals into.

My first question to him was, what was more important, the Ironman or the highly competitive placing in Sprint and Olympic races? He told me the Ironman. I asked why. After thinking for a few minutes, he said, "Because I'm afraid I can't do it." I decided, in that moment of his honesty and clarity, that he was an athlete I would choose to coach. I have learned that when you make a commitment to do something big, it demands a bigger spirit. It creates growth that sometimes is completely unexpected and maybe even scary. Greg knew this already and was brave enough to take on the challenge of the Ironman. I would help him navigate through that growth and encourage him to expand his consciousness.

We started a dialogue about his goals and what the "big rocks" were for him. You may know the story of putting the big rocks in the jar first. If you put in sand, gravel, and small rocks first, there is no room for the big rocks, but when you put the big rocks in first, there is more room than you can imagine for the smaller stuff. He had told me Ironman was his priority, making it the one big rock he wanted to choose. We initially looked ahead and chose a fall race, eight or nine months out from that first meeting, and plotted how that would logistically fit into his life. He considered his daughters, his summer of training, and thought for a few days about what he really wanted. He opted for an early summer Ironman the next year and decided to focus on the shorter distances in the coming race season. Once that big rock was established, we could fill in the smaller rocks and get him on track for a strong race season.

Greg was on the road of awareness and consciousness. He wanted to challenge himself physically and was excited and scared at the same time in choosing his race goals. He understood that he was exploring a potential vulnerability in order to have a profound experience. In daring to take on something so big, he was stepping into an arena of uncertainty with the courage to try. There was no guarantee that he would get to the starting line of Ironman, let alone the finish line. But he had given birth to a desire that, despite the risk, was opening a door to who he really was.

Are you putting the big rocks in your jar first?

Consider things like recovering fully, developing awareness, creating energy credit instead of debt, learning to be mindful, having an attitude of gratitude, and being aligned with your life's purpose. These are the big rocks I suggest you start to look at if you have hit a wall and don't know what to do to perform and live better.

> Are you putting the big rocks in your jar first?

When you are wide awake, conscious, and aware of what you are doing and why, each and every day, you will most certainly show up better in your sport and in your life. By noticing what unconsciousness has already cost you, you have begun the process of changing and moving into that greater person deep inside you.

Where the Trouble Lies

The issue for most of us as human beings—and many of us as athletes—is that we are trained to look only at the surface of things. We develop only a superficial awareness of what we do and why we do it. We may spend years in a sport thinking we are being healthy and fit, and on the surface we look the part, or we hope to compete at elite levels with harder and harder work. The deeper cost of living only on the surface of our bodies may stop us in our tracks at some point. The inability to shine that light on ourselves and figure out what we are really doing will also catch up with us.

Starting to Shift

Susie ran cross country for her high school team. She had natural ability, and her coach encouraged her to tap into that ability. In her freshman year, she rocked the seniors' world by being the fastest female on the team. She ran more miles each year than the previous year, did interval training over each summer, signed up for a plyometric training program offered by a local gym, and obsessed about how to get faster each season. Over those four years, she suffered many injuries, including compartment syndrome, amenorrhea, plantar fasciitis, and chronic patellar pain in her right knee. By the end of her senior year, she was emotionally spent, physically exhausted, and injured beyond the level that she could still race. The colleges that had been interested in her through her sophomore and junior years suddenly had nothing to offer her when she graduated. She was devastated.

Like Susie, many of us need to develop more insight into our own body, mind, and inner being. In a more powerful, penetrating awareness of ourselves and our motivations, we can live a more purposeful and healthy life and redefine possibility. As our big rocks shift, we may have to make room for things we didn't even have to consider before. Susie had to let go of her dream to run in college before she could even begin to accept what new "rock" would come into her life to replace cross country. At first, you may not even know what to do with yourself or that space created when the rock comes out, but with consciousness and patience, you will most likely come to realize that letting go is one of the greatest gifts you can give yourself. If you don't let go, you most certainly will continue to be dragged.

Jeff had been an athlete all his life. He ran track in high school and college and continued into adulthood finding triathlon. Years of pushing himself and being pushed by his coaches brought him high levels of achievement not only athletically but also professionally. Personally, he was not so successful. He seldom talked about the two failed marriages under his belt. He worked hard, pushed his limits, and excelled in his job and his sport. Until he didn't. A trip to the emergency room one summer with severe abdominal pain paired with an out-of-control heart rate during training and racing that same summer required him to pay attention to what his body was telling him and learn how to take time to rest and recover.

Jeff thought he had his life under control. Each year he had set bigger goals, and for a while, he attained them. When he looked back, there were subtle signs before that trip to the emergency room that he ignored or didn't even really notice. His resting heart rate was climbing, his sleep was not as good as it used to be, and it took longer for him to recover from races than it used to. If he had listened to the whispers, his body would not have had to yell.

You can develop awareness at whatever stage of life and sport you are in. Whether you are a young teen hoping to go to college on an athletic scholarship, or a business person looking to stay fit and healthy, coming into a deeper awareness of yourself and your motivations will most certainly help you achieve "success" in this new and broadened definition.

So, you might be thinking, "Where do I start this journey from unconsciousness to becoming a conscious athlete?"

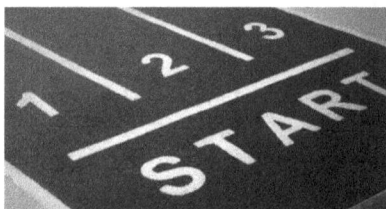

Take a Deep Breath

―――――― ✧ ――――――

Breath is the bridge which connects life to consciousness, which unites your body to your thoughts. Whenever your mind becomes scattered, use your breath as the means to take hold of your mind again.

—Thich Nhat Hanh

―――――― ✧ ――――――

Conscious awareness is as simple as holding a steady focus, and as complicated as holding a steady focus. If you have already been using mindfulness techniques—and especially if you have not—I want you to focus first on the most basic thing you can: your breathing. Control over your breath is control over your life. Breath is the tool that holds the body and mind together. One of the best ways to enter the elusive "zone" when performing is being able to find this calm, confident, relaxed state. Breath is the first step in finding that powerful place by consciously telling our brain that everything is okay, which therefore allows us to access our abilities and higher thinking.

A respiratory center at the base of your brain, in the medulla, controls your breathing. It is part of your Autonomic Nervous System (ANS), which has two parts: the Sympathetic Nervous System (SNS), and the Parasympathetic Nervous System (PNS). The control center will continuously send signals to the respiratory muscles to contract and relax automatically, without any consciousness on your part. The strongest influence on the activity of your breathing center is carbon dioxide (CO_2) levels in your blood and cerebrospinal fluid. When high carbon dioxide levels are detected, your brain says to breathe faster. When your brain detects this increase in respiratory rate, it thinks you are in trouble.

Your breath happens unconsciously, but you do have the ability to consciously control the rate and depth. In taking control of your breathing, you get to tell your brain whether you are in trouble or not. If your brain detects stress by noticing a fast, shallow respiration rate, it goes into a SNS response of fight, flight, or freeze, and dumps adrenaline and cortisol into your body so you can respond to that perceived stress or threat. On the other hand, if your brain detects a slow, deep respiratory rate, it goes into a PNS response of calm, and dumps acetylcholine and DHEA into your body, which help you revitalize.

According to the Bohr Effect, the lower your blood pH and the higher your blood CO_2 levels, the easier it is for your body to "absorb" oxygen. Therefore, if we inhale too early before truly needing to from a physiological standpoint, we're putting a cap on our maximum minute ventilation. In simpler terms, we're maxing out our breathing rate before we have a chance to max out our oxygen absorption. Adding to that, poor CO_2 tolerance is correlated to poor breathing control. Any and all athletes want to have strong breathing muscles and excellent breathing control so that the pulmonary system (i.e. the lungs and surrounding structures) will never be the weak link; lactate threshold and/or movement economy should always be the weak link in endurance performance. (CruxFit, 2019)

If I can get my brain to think I am *not* stressed just by controlling my breath, why wouldn't I? Think about being on the starting line of a big race or the first whistle of your championship game. You are able to be calm, focused, and confident instead of anxious, scattered, and uneasy. Bringing breath into consciousness can do just that.

Try this simple test to measure your CO_2 tolerance:

1. Take four full breaths into your abdomen through your nose: a 3–5 second inhale, followed by a 5–10 second relaxed exhale, one second pause before beginning to inhale again.

2. At the top of the fourth inhale (totally full), start a timer and exhale through your nose as slowly as possible. Stretch out the exhale for as long as possible and sit in the bottom of the breath as long as is comfortable. You may want to close your eyes so that you can stay relaxed.

3. Stop the timer when your air runs out, or you feel the first urge to inhale.

Less than 20 seconds is the low-end score, meaning you have very high anxiety and stress tolerance, 20–40 seconds is average with moderate to high stress and anxiety, 40–60 seconds is intermediate and you can improve quickly with CO_2 tolerance training, 60–80 seconds is advanced and shows good breathing and stress control, and over 80 seconds is elite. The good news is, you can train your CO_2 tolerance with breathing exercises. Simply start by consciously controlling the rate and depth. Sit quietly for 10 minutes while observing and consciously controlling your breathing. Begin by simply making the exhale longer than the inhale, breathing in and out through the nose, feeling your abdomen expand and contract. As you become comfortable with that, add a pause at the top of the breath, and eventually pause also at the bottom.

Box breathing, or 4-4-4-4 breath, is another simple way to begin to teach CO_2 tolerance that you can do any time of the day. Breathe in for four counts, hold for four, breathe out for four, and hold for four.

Our minds jump around and insist that we pay attention to what they choose, not what we choose, unless we practice how to override that impulse to latch onto something new every other moment. Yogis call it monkey mind, like a monkey out of control, swinging from tree to tree. Without strengthening our ability to hold conscious awareness and focus, we are at the mercy of that monkey. Many of us don't notice this very common tendency, because we have a regular pathway of things that grab hold of our attention almost all day, whether it's projects at home or at work, music, TV, reading, our phones, or one conversation after another.

Consciously choosing to hone your focus is very different than just attending to what comes into your realm of attention. If you play a sport that requires a lot of hand-eye coordination and is very dynamic and fluid, being able to follow the game, puck, or ball with complete consciousness will make you a better player, rather than being distracted by things that don't require your attention to score goals or stop goals from being scored on you.

Have you ever been talking to someone who you realize isn't listening to you? They are distracted and somewhere else in their mind. Whether you are on the playing field, at work, or in a relationship, being present and focused is a skill that serves you in all aspects of your life. Learning to focus because you want to be a better athlete will add value to and enhance your life in general.

Steady focus is a skill you can develop at a very small cost and with a very large benefit. Conscious awareness allows you to notice things about your body you might not previously have paid attention to. Listening to the subtle whisper of injury will most certainly reduce the time that you are sidelined rather than waiting for it to yell and cost you a surgery. Sara, who endured years of knee pain, ended up being more defined by her injury than her ability. If you're training with conscious awareness, and notice after a hard strength workout that your left shoulder is sore, you might throw less in your softball practice the next day and find yourself ready to play that weekend instead of sitting out on the injury roster.

A better developed consciousness using breath training allows you to be an observer of your thoughts. When you really listen to your self-talk, you start to understand how much worry or anger you unconsciously allow that keeps you in fear-based behavior rather than consciously moving into confidence-based performance excellence. You might learn to manage not only that fear and anxiety on the playing field, but also in your work and relationships. Hope instead of hopelessness, patience instead of impatience, the glass half full instead of half empty are conscious choices to show up better, regardless of where you are.

Learning to focus on breath yields a steady focus that will give you penetrating insight into yourself and your performance. Such focus leads you to greater moments of awakening, those "Aha, I get it now" moments where quantum leaps can happen. When you are aware, you can really see what you are doing well, and what you need to work on. In seeing what you need to work on, you can decide whether you need help with better coaching, or whether you can make the adjustments and corrections yourself. Learning to swing a golf club to drive the ball further may be something you can teach yourself, but taking a look at why you throw that club every time you don't hit the ball as far as you would like may require some outside help.

The Bigger Picture

Consciousness can be part of your training plan like any other skill in sport necessary for you to work on. Learning to listen to your body is often something you are not taught or even encouraged to ignore:

> "Stop whining."
> "Don't be a baby."
> "No pain, no gain."
> "What does not kill you makes you stronger."

Who among us has not heard that at some point in our athletic lives? It is true that you do have to work hard and push yourself to see results, but not at the expense of an injury to your body and your confidence. If you have hip pain after a 10-mile run on Saturday, and you show up at track practice Wednesday morning, still in pain but dulling it with anti-inflammatories, that whisper of injury may have to become a scream in order to come into your awareness enough for you to address it. Too many of us pride ourselves on pushing through pain rather than paying attention to it. Missing one track practice may stop an injury that has the potential to put you in physical therapy for months, sideline you for a season, or even take you out of your sport for the rest of your life.

Becoming more aware in your life may also have long-term benefits you have not considered before. If your sport takes you away from your family and your responsibilities, you may want to actually listen to your spouse when they complain you are never home on the weekends. If you schedule your relationship time with as much awareness as your training time, over the long run, it may not just keep you out of divorce court, but also improve your marriage.

Choosing your race season based on your son's baseball schedule or your daughter's swim meets will tell the most important people in your life that you care about them more than your sport. No sport is worth losing people you love and who love you. I tell all my athletes who are stepping up to Ironman distance training or to the next level of competition in whatever sport they participate in that there are no divorces on my watch. Families have to be on board with the decision to take on that kind of commitment and be aware of what the training will require and cost them.

Having a higher consciousness can also help you deal with an outcome in sport that is different than you had expected. In understanding that there are no failures, only opportunities and invitations to learn, you might always discover your potential not just in winning, but in how you deal with loss and what you learn from it.

David came to me looking for a coach after his life had collapsed under him. He was searching for some solid ground to stand on. Who he had been for 45 years had suddenly changed. The athlete in him was the first place he looked to find stability. He had run several marathons already and decided that Ironman training was a place where he might find some calm in the storm of his life. He was not unconscious and had no delusions as to why he took on the challenge, and it just may have helped him to save his sanity.

He put in countless hours of training, especially in the pool, where he determined he actually had such poor ankle flexibility that he joked that he went backwards when he kicked. We found a bike for him that he could afford and set it up so it didn't hurt his neck that had been injured years ago. He was fiercely moving towards a more authentic self and life, and Ironman training helped.

Race day arrived. He bravely stepped up to the starting line of Ironman Lake Placid. Despite losing his goggles and watch in the swim, he made it to the bike. He missed the cutoff time for the bike course after a derailleur issue that threw his chain more times than he could count. Knowing his strength was the run, and that he could have easily completed those 26.2 miles, he accepted the end of his day and enjoyed the next few hours with his three children who were there cheering him on and supporting him.

David was not disappointed in not finishing the race. He was aware and conscious enough already to be grateful for that time he got to spend with his children, sharing his experience and understanding of what was really important in his life: family and the journey. Gifts often come wrapped in different packages than we expect. We only have to be open enough to receive them. Crossing the finish line is not always the gift race day offers us. Getting to the starting line and accepting what the day had to offer were the gifts David was given that day, and he received them with complete grace.

Your Current Mindset May Be Your Biggest Obstacle

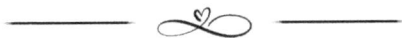

It is easy to get discouraged while doing benevolent work, as the outcome of our efforts may not be immediately apparent.

—The Daily Om

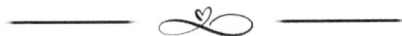

Like any other skill in sport, consciousness can be practiced. You can develop and strengthen your awareness just like any muscle in your body. As in anything we learn, there are obstacles you might encounter in the process. Having a mind that is not yet harnessed will most certainly be one of those obstacles. Being hyper-focused on outcome certainly breeds competitiveness and frustration if you don't always win. You may be your own biggest obstacle, because you are already resisting this premise. You believe that hard work and winning are what is most important. You scoff at self-analysis and "the journey" as New Age crap.

Years ago, I went to watch my son coach a U-11 boys' lacrosse team at a tournament on one of the hottest weekends of the summer. These youngsters played hard, listened to their coaches and their parents, and, from my perspective, did their best. They made it to the playoffs in a game that would give them either third or fourth place in the tournament. I overheard one of the other coaches say, "We are playing for second loser."

What an absolute tragedy.

With such complete unawareness of the opportunity to help these boys develop their own consciousness and strengthen their love of the game, that coach was *not* one I would have liked my son to have been playing for when he was 11. He was disappointed at what he perceived to be a loss and projected that into the situation, unaware of what he could teach those players about perseverance, endurance, positive attitude, or sportsmanship—the things a conscious, athlete-centered coach would know how to do.

Like everything in life that is worthwhile, learning to become conscious takes time. You will probably not be good at this new skill at first, and that will either frustrate you or inspire you. You get to choose. It will also take patience. Learning to kick a field goal is a measurable skill and when you practice, you can measure when the ball goes further. The need to see immediate evidence of progress can be the most significant hindrance to building consciousness. We want results from our practice and we want them quickly. Practicing conscious awareness with its slow increase in results may be counterintuitive to the unaware athlete that expects change to happen fast.

Developing a consciousness and awareness of yourself requires time, patience, and persistence. It is easier to get discouraged or dismissive than it is to be patient or confident that things are shifting when the outcome of our efforts may not be apparent as quickly or as visibly as we would like. Heck, for me, patience is a practice I was not born with, let alone consciousness. I have had to practice patience even more than awareness. Change is never easy, but it is always worth it.

"Absent-Bodyness" Syndrome

The physical body gets a lot of attention because we know it, can measure it, and we can see improvement. Even with all the focus we put on our bodies, there is an "absent-bodiedness" syndrome I see where we live far outside the walls of our bodies and ignore it when it needs our attention the most. In absent-mindedness, we operate without thinking; in absent-bodiedness, we operate without listening to or being present in our bodies. Because of that, most of us have, at some point, overdone physical activity and ended up injured, ill, or simply burned out.

Can you even imagine working your consciousness to that point? The funny thing is that, often, what directs our attention to consciousness is exactly the crisis that forces us to slow down or maybe even stop. It is often the unconscious mind that leads us down the path of destruction and allows us, if we are ready, to come into consciousness and learn new ways to build constructive, healthy alignment in our lives. Our broken down bodies, unsuccessful relationships, and our lives wandering off course are passageways, vehicles, on the necessary road to consciousness.

The Inside Out Approach

If you are looking to improve your performance and increase your conscious awareness, this book will guide you.

Focus on and consider these questions:

- How do you plug into attitudes and beliefs about yourself and your life?
- How do you think you will change the attitudes and beliefs that need to be changed?
- Do you even want to make these changes?

It is not easy to be conscious of our weaknesses, to focus on them, and then to work towards making them strengths. Beginning the process of looking inward rather than outward may take you outside of your comfort zone. When you lack awareness, there is a disconnect. Behavior is very goal-oriented when there is an external focus on outcome or some measurement of performance. Sport can be used as an escape, an excuse, a pacifier, or a drug to keep awareness at bay. Sometimes the biggest overachievers are the most self-loathing. What we are achieving has less to do with who we are and more to do with proving who we are not. Shining the light inside you, exposing thoughts, behaviors, beliefs and attitudes, or dark places you have been avoiding or unaware of may be extremely uncomfortable, but it will take you to new heights in your performance and in your life.

The inside out approach may seem like "belly button staring," but my experience is that a lot of belly buttons conceal a lot of issues. We often use methods to avoid investigating the depths of who we are—methods like alcohol, affairs, drugs, and yes, even exercise. When we compete, there is no way for our inner issues not to affect our performance and outcome. It is better to address those issues, own them, and use them in a positive way, rather than a negative and obsessive way. Addiction always ends badly and limits us as athletes and as human beings.

If you are focusing on the external or the outcome, you most certainly have a diminished awareness of what is going on inside you. As you step up to this new starting line of awareness/consciousness, you may feel the same nervousness, uncertainty, and doubt as you did at your first event. You are about to venture into something new, unknown, unfamiliar. You may wonder what difference it will make or how it will fit into that canvas of your life. Just as you had to practice the physical skills demanded in your sport, you will have to practice consciousness. You may learn that practice is a virtue and perfection is not as important as progress.

When you practice consciousness, you have the ability to give birth to something deep inside of you that has been waiting to come out. Something that is authentic, passionate, enthusiastic, and powerful. Practicing conscious awareness teaches you to change your thoughts, to choose your emotions, and to manage your time and energy. In that deeper dive into yourself, you may be uncertain where you are headed and uncomfortable in the depths. I can promise that what you discover there will be worth it. When you reveal your highest self and highest potential, you no longer have to live in a false image you created for yourself or others. There will be no more need to pretend to be someone you believe is better than the person you really are. You may discover that there is an athlete inside you capable of more than you know. You may even discover that "athlete" is a stepping stone to revealing more about who you are than you can imagine.

Perhaps the real purpose behind taking on the physical challenges we do is to find enlightenment, meaning, purpose. We simply have not looked beyond the physical yet, or don't even know how.

4

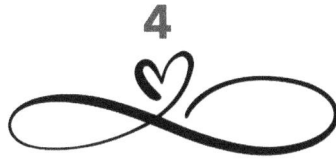

The Missing Piece: Consciousness

Are you an athlete looking for the latest technology or training methodology, nutrition plan, or coach? Or perhaps a better training environment or secret that only the professionals know to enhance your performance? If you have been looking *outside* yourself and have yet to look *inside* yourself to improve your game or get faster, you may find it after reading this book.

As we have already discussed in the previous chapters, there is something already inside and accessible to you that you might not even know exists. It is such a powerful, yet underrated tool and is already operating on its own without your awareness. Unharnessed, this power may be exactly what is stopping you from achieving the success you want. It may be working against you, rather than for you, until you learn to use it to your advantage.

That power is, simply and profoundly, *consciousness*.

As easy as that sounds, as daring as it can be to come into fuller awareness, looking inward to the skills that consciousness offers is the way to reach new potential—perhaps your highest potential.

So, what do I mean by consciousness?

Recall that the concept of consciousness is often attributed to John Locke. He defined consciousness as the *perception* of what passes in a man's own mind.

What is most important about Locke's statement is that he was pointing to the fact that we as humans have the ability to *observe* and be *aware* of what is passing through our minds rather than just allowing our thoughts, and the deeper, unconscious beliefs and feelings that drive them, to pass through us unattended. By attending to and paying attention to our thoughts, we have the ability and power to observe our own mind, and to harness and influence it for good use.

We have the ability to not only change our perception of what passes through our minds, but to also decide *what* passes through.

Why is that skill of observation, which can intentionally be developed, so important to athletes?

Our minds are powerful tools. Becoming aware of and curious about what passes through your mind while consciously choosing what enhances your performance, will allow you to make profound changes at a whole new level and to find possibilities you might never have even dreamed of.

We all have a stream of continuous thought that goes through our minds, like a ticker tape moving constantly with all kinds of information. If you could download it at the end of the day and read it, you might wonder, "Who is that inside my head talking like that?" Michael Singer, in his book *The Untethered Soul*, calls it "the roommate in your head." (Singer, 2007) If you had a roommate that talked to you like that, you would probably evict them. Singer tells us that we are not that thinking mind, we are the consciousness behind that mind and are aware of those thoughts. Our consciousness has the ability to focus in a sharp, narrow way or expand to a broader perspective depending on what is best for us to pay attention to at any given moment. It is a dynamic field of awareness you can tap into. You and your consciousness run the show, not the thoughts.

Our mind is simply the place where our thoughts reside; your mind "thinks." Left to its own devices, it is unsupervised constant noise and chatter. Without harnessing our thoughts, we don't have the opportunity to be conscious of what passes through our minds. If your mind is not under your control, you may be living a life that your mind "thinks," rather than what you choose to think. Learning to control and harness your thoughts, your emotions, your true self, and practicing new skills that may initially be counterintuitive to you are the ways to use what is inside you to change not only your performance, but your life.

Just as you had to practice all the skills necessary for your sport physically, you will have to practice all these mindfulness or mental and emotional skills. You understand that swinging a bat over and over again will make you a better baseball player. Now you will understand that just as practicing your swing, practicing new thoughts, choosing what emotions you feel, breathing with awareness, and increasing your ability to focus will also make you better at your sport.

There is a small, quiet voice, an intuition, a knowing that is inside of us all that needs space in your mind and heart to be heard and felt. Learning to open the door to that voice and close the doors on the roommate may just help you achieve more in your sport and your life than you could ever have imagined.

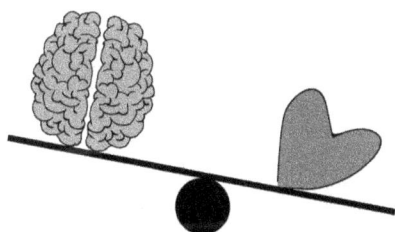

The skills of consciousness are important to learn. They allow a deeper knowing of who we are and what we are capable of through innate wisdom. Consciousness in sport allows us to tap into, to find that awareness, and to live authentically with it. When we consciously compete with acute awareness of ourselves and our environment, we can acquire that wisdom. We may not innately possess those skills, but we can most certainly learn them.

In his book *Power vs Force*, author David Hawkins tells us,

> The truth be told, all human endeavors have the common goal of understanding or influencing human experience. Regardless of what arena of inquiry one starts from: philosophy, political theory, theology, psychology, or even sport, all quests for understanding eventually converge at a common meeting point: *the quest for an organized understanding of the nature of pure consciousness.* (Hawkins, 2013)

My belief, based on my experience as a coach and athlete, is that *a better developed state of consciousness* is the missing component in sports training programs today. It's my personal mission to add this to the athlete's spectrum of training.

The Question

Years ago, in one of my first-aid exams for a coaching certification, there was a question I found obvious at the time, but actually believe to be quite profound. Little did I know that I would be looking at consciousness as a state of awareness rather than simply a medical condition. The question said:

When dealing with an unconscious athlete, the first action that must be taken is:

A. Roll the athlete onto their back.
B. Stop any bleeding that may be severe.
C. *Determine the level of consciousness and unresponsiveness.*
D. Check the athlete's carotid pulse.

Notice that we need to determine the level of consciousness and unresponsiveness before we proceed with any other life-saving—or in this case, performing-enhancing—action.

Let's figure out where you are on this spectrum of consciousness and move you towards a deeper understanding of yourself and your motivation for why you participate in sport. At this point, you may want to take some time to get a clearer understanding of where you are now physically, mentally, emotionally, and spiritually. Perhaps you will begin to see what is missing and how to find it for yourself. The journey towards greater awareness and insight will be a most personal one. There are no right or wrong answers, only ones that are open and honest.

Why is it necessary to be clear about where we stand physically, mentally, emotionally, and spiritually?

It's because consciousness allows depth, and depth gives us a stronger foundation for fitness and athleticism than focusing only on the physical aspect of our being. Not incidentally, depth matters in all the rest of life, too. We can recall certain days in fine detail—maybe days our children were born, days we traveled and saw something spectacular, days we lost someone we loved or days of intense emotion, as well as days we competed. We remember because we were conscious, aware, connected. And then there are days that go by when we don't even know where we were or what we were doing. Becoming conscious connects us more to life, how we live it, and brings what is important into our awareness.

In any sport, there is a lot going on inside and out when you compete and perform. By deliberately paying more attention to and choosing what is going on inside of you and your body, there is unlimited potential to have the inside enhance your performance. External chaos is a given every time we compete. Learning to not react to it and bring it inside us is where the real power lies. Learning that we may not be able to control our environment, but we can control how we deal with that environment is key. Stress comes when we "think" we should be able to change things we cannot. It is that "thinking" that takes us out of our ability to perform at our best and into a mode of negative reactiveness.

Awareness: Why is This Skill So Important?

In acknowledging that you could be more aware, you will be able to take the first step towards consciousness. Awareness allows us to show up better in life. It harnesses our minds' ability to monitor and analyze our own thoughts, our internal being, and our external environment. By learning to focus on the internal being, you can develop a deep knowledge of yourself and gain control of your thoughts and your emotions. When you are aware, you are not using activity as a distraction, but as a way to find purpose, meaning, and alignment in life. If you think of awareness as a flashlight that pierces through the veils of illusions we have unconsciously bought into and illuminates the reality that is behind those veils, you can see how you develop a kind of clarity or sobriety in your life, rather than being intoxicated by emotions and fear. Emotions can show you the parts of yourself operating outside of your awareness if you are willing to look at them. It does not require genius, only that you become a curious observer.

1. Take a deep breath in and out.
2. Begin to notice what you feel.
3. Take note of the thoughts moving through your mind.
4. How do you act or react to those feelings and thoughts?
5. What are the consequences or rewards of those actions and reactions in your life?

When you start to listen to your intuition, pay attention to what you are perceiving, open your eyes to a new reality, then you will start to lift those veils of illusion you have been living behind and move into a more real and authentic life. Your consciousness is raised along with the frequency of your thoughts.

To make conscious choices, ask yourself three questions and have the perseverance to find the answers.

1. Why am I doing this sport?
2. What do I really want from this sport?
3. How do I bring the why and the want into greater alignment?

You can find the answers to those questions by learning to increase your awareness. All athletes know how to work hard. It's a matter of taking that same work ethic into a new realm of understanding and practice—one of looking inside.

We all have some understanding of who we are. There are measures of self that are ingrained deeply in our consciousness that may have more to do with what someone else told us about ourselves than what we know to be true based on our own wisdom. Finding and releasing illusions we have bought into can be, for many of us, the key to finding our real but hidden power and passion. The beliefs we have that operate under our radar of knowing are simply chronic patterns of thought that we learned when we were young. Just like we can change a chronic, learned pattern of movement that no longer serves us in our lives, or resulted in some kind of injury to our body, we can change those patterns of thought that have resulted in limiting our potential.

This work is really about who you *are*, not who you *think* you are. It's about being able to clear the view of yourself that has been clouded with limiting beliefs so that you can fully realize and access the real self that has been there all along. We grow up being told what to do, what we are good at, how to behave; are rewarded for some behaviors and punished for others. Fitting into a mold that someone else builds for us often makes us contortionists or conformists rather than vibrant and authentic human beings.

As you start to practice your new skill set—or, as I like to call it, a tool-box with tools better suited to your new consciousness—you will learn to examine your choices, your life, and answer some hard questions you may not have considered before.

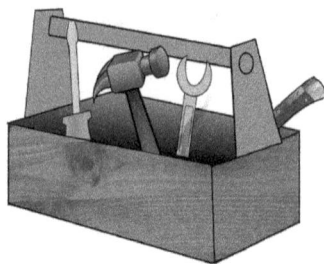

When athletes I have coached have come into fuller consciousness, they often talk about having a sense that something had been missing or that they felt something was lost somewhere inside them or in their lives. Becoming more conscious was the way they found what they were really looking for. Bringing yourself more fully into your training and your performance is what I hope you are looking for—and find—from reading this book.

The Time of the Conscious Athlete

As the years and decades have passed, I have watched sport grow in many wonderful ways. Friendships have developed, races and tournaments have become annual pilgrimages, families compete together and support each other, technology has improved, and the science of sport has taken off. There are new governing bodies, studies of technique, the body and of the brain; records are broken every day and limits are questioned regarding what we are capable of as human beings.

I have also watched as athletes learned to disregard their intuition. They remain unconscious and instead choose to listen outside themselves: their coach, nutritionist, power meter, heart rate monitor, pros, or the latest post on a chat room. It is true that all those things may help you improve in your sport and attain your goals, but consciousness is not only about your athletic being—it's about your *whole* being.

Today, it's time for the emergence of the conscious athlete—the one who is acutely tuned to their whole being.

I say this because, today, we witness parents sending their young children to "experts" who promise to build young champions with training programs better suited to more developed bodies that are conditioned to endure the higher training intensities they deem necessary to excel. Unnecessary injuries are happening in elementary, middle, and high schools that take young athletes out of sport for the rest of their lives, most often because parents and coaches are pushing a process that promises immediate results rather than grooming their children and athletes in a way that is consistent with not only their physical development, but also their own desires and passions.

Some coaches and trainers work with athletes in a way that serves the athlete, and then there are coaches who work in ways that serve themselves. When you work with anyone to help you achieve goals, be sure that the goals are your own and not those of someone who uses you to serve their program or gym or reputation. An athlete-centered program recognizes moral development, health, and education of all athletes as essential requirements in the pursuit of excellence. Look for coaches that build confidence, see possibility instead of limits, and understand the value of effort and learning along with improved performance. Trainers and coaches who commit to the improvement of the individual athlete—where the focus is on the athlete's needs and not on the coach's agendas—are building conscious athletes rather than unthinking, obedient ones. Joe Ehrmann and Gregory Jordan, in their book *InSideOut Coaching,* refer to these coaches as "transformational." Ehrmann writes about how he used his football career as a "lifelong, often desperate search for acceptance and approval from adults who had power and authority over me." He calls these coaches "transactional… [they] use players as tools to meet their personal needs for validation, status, and identity." (Ehrmann and Jordan, 2011)

Athlete-centered, coach-driven programs encourage you to uncover what you already possess; to be pulled toward growth and grounded in self-direction. These programs encourage intuition and self-awareness, and the coaches actually listen to their athletes. Beware of coaches that are at the center of their programs and use their athletes to drive them. They tend to be about pushing and forcing change, most times at the expense of their athletes. The Canadian Sport for Life Model and John O'Sullivan's Changing the Game Project are places for you to look if you are the parent of a young athlete or you were coached in your own youth by someone who had their best interests at heart instead of yours. The approach of raising happy, high-performing athletes and giving sport back to our youth is one truly in alignment with the message of this book.

Training in the area of awareness and personal growth is generally not taught, and is what I intend to offer you with the lessons from this book. You may learn to embrace adversity and focus more on what you can control, rather than be upset about what you cannot. Seeing what is possible, committing to removing your blind spots, taking responsibility for self-imposed barriers, and preparing to move out of the performance arena into the bigger arena of your life—these are the things a good coach will help teach you.

Not only is it the time of the conscious athlete, it's also the time of the conscious coach.

With the right environment, support, and deeper consciousness, you will become a better athlete and you may even find yourself showing up better in all areas of your life.

How Conscious Are You?

It's my observation that athletes often don't know or don't want to look at why they do what they do. They may spend countless hours working toward their measurable goals. They spend time on sport-specific skills in the gym, on the yoga mat, in the chiropractor's office, at physical therapy, on the massage table, online looking at the latest equipment and attire. When you commit that much time, energy, money, and thought to one aspect of your being, why would you not also develop a good understanding of what it is that drives you toward that aspect of your life?

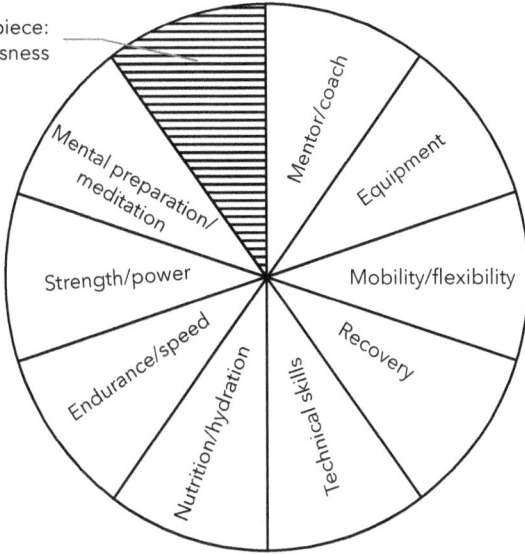

The missing piece: Consciousness

Mentor/coach
Equipment
Mobility/flexibility
Recovery
Technical skills
Nutrition/hydration
Endurance/speed
Strength/power
Mental preparation/meditation

Have you looked inwardly at the motivation behind how you live your life? Do you really understand what gets you out of bed each morning to get your workout in before work? Do you look at the thoughts and emotions that pass through your own mind? Are the choices you make an action of living consciously or are they a reaction, a way to cope with an unfulfilled life?

I invite you to look at the chart below and consider where you fall on the continuum of awareness.

EXTERNAL FOCUS	INTERNAL FOCUS
Increased focus on outcome Decreased awareness	Decreased focus on outcome Increased awareness
Force	Power/Feel
Heart rate/Watts/Mph	Lessons
Pace/Time	Flow/Joy
Placing/Score	Resonance/Authenticity

If you are more focused on the score of your game rather than what the event and the training has to teach you *regardless of outcome*, you might consider looking deeper at your motivations and bringing these traits more into balance.

If you know how much power you can produce at your lactate threshold heart rate, how fast you can throw a ball, or what your vertical jump is, but you have no idea how it feels to be there without the technology in front of you telling you, I can assure you there is some new learning ahead—a skill that can teach you to listen to your body rather than merely training "by the numbers." Numbers can only get you so far. When your mind is clogged with data and over-focused on external factors, you cannot be aware of your internal factors.

If you watch your heart rate monitor every workout and use it as a marker of your improved fitness, that is a great tool to map measurable improvement. If you are not recording and journaling what you learned from those workouts along with your heart rate, however, I can tell you there is room for growth as an athlete and a person. Pace, time, and heart rate are important things for athletes to know; learning what it means to be in the flow of a sport, finding joy, and being open to the lessons it teaches can take you to its next level.

When you shift your awareness from the outside to the inside, there is no doubt that you will discover pieces of yourself you didn't even know existed. When you step up to a starting line or onto a playing field with these new pieces, you have the capacity to be more present and engaged. When you are observing and directing your thoughts and your feelings, you are in a place of authenticity, awareness, and as a result, are more powerful.

You will have found resonance when you live your life from a place of authenticity, when who you are and what you want out of life are in alignment with what you are doing. When you can show up on the playing field excited and open, allowing the authentic you to compete, you find purpose in who you are, rather than remaining in the fear of who you are not.

Driven or Motivated?

We all have a purpose. In *The Purpose Driven Life*, Rick Warren reminds us that everyone's life is driven by something. You are here for a reason and are part of an intricate plan. (Warren, 2002). That drive could be fear, guilt, the need for approval, anger, or an unconscious belief. Those forces lead to the dead ends of an unfulfilled life, unnecessary stress, and unachieved potential. Lives may have motion but no meaning. We seem to sweat our entire lives on an endless treadmill, seeking a cure for those unhealthy drives with athletic achievement. Without awareness, your life may be driven by fear. By coming into consciousness, your life can be driven by knowing your purpose. It will be simple: you won't need motivation or reward, and you will find passion and meaning.

Some of us move with intention towards fulfilling that purpose, while others wander, not knowing where they are headed or what they are supposed to be doing. Sport allows us to focus in on a purpose, a meaning, a definable measure of our potential, what we are capable of, and what is possible. Accomplishment in some of our minds may somehow equate to a sense of purpose, but in reality, it can merely be ego puffing us up in a competitive way against others who may have no idea why they are competing, either. When you are participating in sport with passion and enthusiasm and using it as a way to develop your purpose in life, you will be engaging with sport as I'm suggesting:

A way to live a deeper, more purposeful, joyful life.

You must have the attitudes found in the beginner's mind and an open heart. Coming into consciousness requires commitment, courage, and self-responsibility so you can move forward in your search for self and purpose. It is a daunting task requiring complete focus and a willingness to confront the uncomfortable and struggle in it. You will build an inner integrity that allows you to let go of lesser goals in favor of greater ones and participate whole-heartedly in performing in and developing your full potential as an athlete and human being.

Jack was a perfect example of a beginner's mind, open hearted, and hopeful that anything was possible. He came to me initially to lose weight for a cruise he was going on. His first workout, he arrived with the biggest coffee I have ever seen. I asked him where his water was and he said, "This coffee is made from water." And so began the journey from non-athletic couch potato with a high-stress job to an Ironman finish line. Jack lost those 40 pounds, started drinking water, and one day asked me if I thought he could do an Ironman in a year. I asked him if he wanted to, and he said yes, would I help him? I told him I would, although he had to make some significant lifestyle changes. He didn't know how to swim, didn't own a bike, and couldn't last five minutes on a treadmill. What he did know was that he wanted to feel better in his body, commit to a goal he was intimidated by, and trusted me to help him. The night before the race, after months of training with epic struggles and epic growth, Jack gave me a card and thanked me for believing in him in a way no one had ever done before. It was one of my favorite moments as a coach to have been part of such a huge trans-formation. Training for Ironman had changed his life in a way nothing else could have. He crossed that finish line with the biggest smile, his young daughter holding his hand, his wife cheering and stepped into a potential he never knew he had.

Recognizing and understanding what drives you is necessary to become a conscious athlete. Paying attention to your thoughts and emotions, what passes through your mind and heart, and understanding that your mind and spirit are more powerful than your body are keys to enhance your experience, your performance, and your life.

Prepare to Start: Ease on Down the Road to Consciousness

The road to consciousness is a simple one in many ways, but for most, it is not always easy. To travel that road, you will have to get stronger in ways you may have never imagined. Some steps will be straightforward, others will be more difficult. You will find obstacles along the way and, as an athlete, you will have to practice things you might not have ever considered before.

If you are looking to go to the next level as an athlete and a person, you must start to expand your vision and your awareness of what is really going on around you and inside you. Most of us look for change from the outside in. Real change starts from the inside out.

When you start to use new skills that allow you to look at your body from the inside out, begin observing thoughts and emotions and breathing consciously, you start down a road of alignment, power, and authenticity; full of potential, satisfaction, and tremendous opportunity in your sport and in your life.

With these new skills, what seems impossible for you right now—in your sport and in your life —really can become possible.

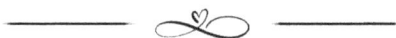

In the end, it is important to remember
we cannot become what we need to be
by remaining what we are.

—Max De Pree, *Leadership Is An Art*

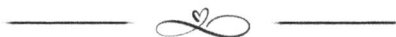

5

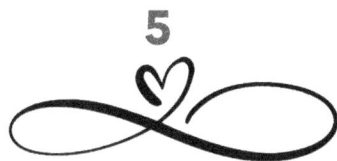

It's Your Move: Conscious Competence

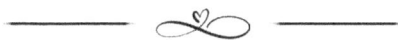

---

*Until you make the unconscious conscious,
it will direct your life, and you will call it fate.*

—Carl Jung

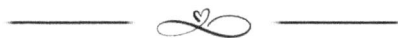

Sport can be a medium that allows us to express ourselves to our fullest potential and, when approached from a new perspective, to realize who we are really meant to be. You can practice steps towards consciousness and begin the journey to yourself where there is no finish line or outcome. More importantly, it's an opportunity to explore, to be who you are and, perhaps in doing so, to fulfill your life's purpose.

It's true that you can have a certain sense of self because of your accomplishments in sport. You might be able to say, "I'm a gold medalist," or "I'm on a team that won three championships," or "I just ran my personal best in the marathon." Because you identify with the sport you compete in, you might define yourself as a gymnast or a hockey player.

But it is equally important to develop a strong, healthy self apart from sport regardless of what you have accomplished. When you can disconnect from outcomes and know who you are outside of your sport, you have a strong foundation for achieving high performance—and also, as it happens, to create a life of fulfillment, happiness, and purpose.

The fact is, we are human *beings*, not human *doings*. We are both body and mind. As healthy physical growth comes from exercising our bodies, healthy conscious growth comes from exercising our minds in all of their dimensions.

Learning Conscious Competence

To move towards consciousness requires the acknowledgement that, at a minimum, you could benefit from being more aware and more intuitive. Awareness is the ability of the mind to monitor and analyze our internal being and external environment. Intuition is instinctive knowledge: the state of being aware of or knowing something without having to discover or perceive it. With awareness and intuition, you can develop a deep knowledge of yourself. You can learn to have control of your thoughts and emotions and, as a result, make conscious choices in your life.

Becoming conscious is just like becoming faster, fitter, leaner, stronger, better at whatever skills your sport demands. It takes a willingness to learn new skills and a dedicated practice of those skills. The same way we practice neuromuscular patterns to lay down the correct technique that our sport requires, we also create neural patterns that lay down thought and emotion patterns in our brain. The same way exercise sculpts our bodies, thoughts and feelings sculpt our minds and hearts.

When we are so good at something that we don't even have to think, when it has become second nature, we say, "It's just like riding a bike. Once you learn, you never forget." There was a time when you didn't know how to ride a bike and you had to learn. Just as there is no way to learn how to ride a bike without getting on it, there is no way to become conscious without looking inside yourself. The first time on your bike, you didn't know how to balance on two small wheels; the first time you take a look inside, you won't know what you are supposed to be looking for.

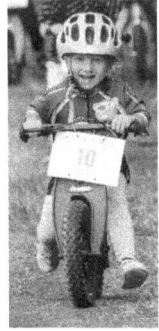

There is a theory of learning called "conscious competence" that perhaps has origins as old as Confucius and Socrates. It is often attributed to the Gospel Guardian article by Martin Broadwell, (Broadwell, 1969), to Noel Burch of Gordon Training International, and W. Lewis Robinson of the International Correspondence Schools.

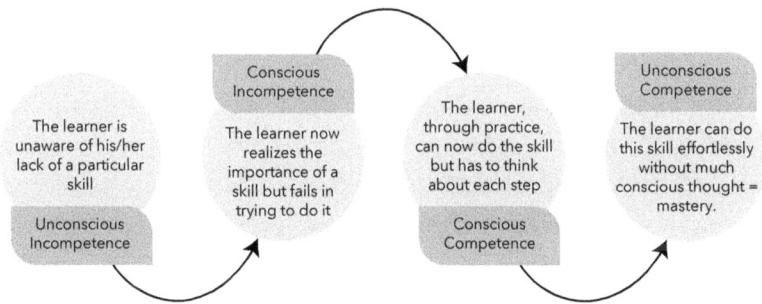

Conscious Incompetence

The learner now realizes the importance of a skill but fails in trying to do it

The learner, through practice, can now do the skill but has to think about each step

Unconscious Competence

The learner can do this skill effortlessly without much conscious thought = mastery.

The learner is unaware of his/her lack of a particular skill

Unconscious Incompetence

Conscious Competence

The Conscious Competence Learning Model
The way we acquire a new skill

The model describes four distinct phases to learning any new skill. It suggests that people are initially naive or unaware of how little they know and are unconscious of their incompetence in that skill. This first stage is referred to as *unconsciously unskilled/incompetent.* A beginner's mind is of value at this stage, regardless of ability. You don't know what you don't know yet, a state of ignorance. Discovery is a big part of the process. Not knowing how to balance, or even to steer, may become evident the first time you ride your bike. Training wheels or no pedals are often used to help develop other skills first. Focusing on the benefits of learning the skill rather than the process of learning will help move through this stage.

As you recognize your incompetence, you have an increased awareness that something is lacking and are now *consciously unskilled/ incompetent.* You know what you *don't know.* This is the most difficult stage, where mistakes must be made in order for learning to begin, where the most patience is required, and where the most judgments against self are formed. As a result, it is also the stage during which most people *give up.* The amount of time you spend here, and whether or not you actually learn the new skill you are now aware of depends on how determined you are to learn it and how you perceive the "failures" while learning it. Being able to overcome discouragement and asking for help at this stage will improve the chances of success. Here, if you start to take inventory of yourself, you may be able to take yourself out of your own way.

Stephanie was a great high school cross-country runner who wanted to run track her senior year. She went out for the team expecting to have the same success and recognition she had running the previous three years. There was no room for error and a mental intensity in the shorter races on the track that she had not experienced in cross-country. She had trouble learning to deal with those new factors. She lasted two track meets and gave up after struggling with the fierce judgment she had of herself in not performing to her expectations. Knowing what she needed to do but not knowing how to do it gave her an opportunity to learn from her mistakes; she did not take this opportunity. She chose to quit instead of using "failure" to progress to the next level of awareness and competence.

Peter wanted to take up tennis at the age of 40. He had played racquetball and figured another game with a racquet and a ball would be easy. His first time on the tennis court was enlightening and humbling. The ball moved at a different speed, the racquet was completely different in size and how it connected to the ball, and he had no walls to work with. He had no idea what he didn't know about the game, and as a result, never stepped back on the court. The initial stage of unconscious incompetence stopped him in his inability to deal with not being "good" at tennis. Peter did not want to look at his inability to learn something new.

When the training wheels come off, or the pedals go on, there may be a few crashes. Those crashes may be perceived as failures that become obstacles to progressing or opportunities to figure out how not to fall. How your brain processes negative experiences will significantly affect how much pain they cause you. Your ability to perceive and recognize the keys to becoming skilled will determine how quickly you are able to move through this stage. If you understand that your mind is just information the nervous system moves (most often outside your awareness), you can use that flow of information or thoughts and feelings to influence and sculpt neural pathways that encourage a calm, happy central nervous system that forms new circuits and strengthens or weakens existing ones easily and quickly.

Becoming *consciously skilled/competent* requires deliberate practice with a degree of thought and effort. You *know* how to do it, but don't know how to do it *yourself* yet. You are learning. You have to be very mindful of what you are doing, but you may still be somewhat uncomfortable and self-conscious. You may be able to ride your bike around your driveway with comfort, but when you move out onto the road with its potholes, curbs, up hills and down hills, you will have to pay more attention to not fall off. There is conscious skill acquisition and then conscious use of that skill. Here is where you improve and know that it starts to show. You dedicate yourself to improvement with repeated practice, participation in more formal training, or you look for someone to coach or mentor you.

If you continue to practice and apply the new skills you learn, you will eventually find that those same skills you didn't even know you needed in the beginning are now easier, perhaps have even become a natural part of you that doesn't require thought. Burch calls it *unconsciously skilled/competent.* The unconsciously competent athlete completes tasks and executes skills with grace, speed, and mastery without thought or concentration. Skills become intuitive and second nature. Riding a bike will eventually become "just like riding a bike."

Learning to become conscious will require moving through those same learning phases. At first, you may not realize that you *are* unconscious to many aspects of yourself. When you know and admit that you are unconscious, you still don't know *how* to become more aware. If you can pass through that difficult stage, you become aware of what you need to do, but won't be good at it yet. Becoming competent at consciousness will come with determination and dedicated practice. Eventually, you may find yourself someday having the ability to have awareness that is as second nature to you as riding a bike.

Some suggest that there is a fifth level of becoming consciously aware of what has been mastered. When you are here, there is the presumption that there is no perfection, that you can always improve, tweak, or fine-tune the skill and then explain it to others to help them achieve it. To be at this fifth level requires an acceptance of personal limitations and openness to learning. You know that you don't know everything. It is a mature practice that requires self-study and self-awareness. There is a constant consciousness of what unconscious abilities are being used, along with constant analysis, adaptation, and augmentation of the skills. It has been called "conscious excellence." If you are riding your bike in a criterium race, you don't want to be on automatic. You choose to be aware of every aspect of your performance. You are very present, very conscious, and use that awareness to analyze and adapt to all the elements of your performance. At this level, you are also able to teach and explain it to others. To me, this sounds very much like the zone—a level of awareness in which we are able to perform at peak in the moment and where we have the powerful and optimal ability to allow opportunity to present itself and meet the circumstance with our highest degree of skill. It requires not only a conscious choice, but also a relaxed and focused mind.

At this point in your athletic career and in your life, whatever point that may be, seriously consider this most difficult stage of which Burch speaks—that of conscious incompetence. The reason it is difficult for most of us is that all learning takes place on the edge of discomfort. Because we are wired neurologically to survive, when something causes you pain or discomfort, your brain is programmed to move away from it or avoid it. As an athlete, you already know that training at intense levels can be very uncomfortable and you have learned how to override the programming and accept that discomfort as necessary to improve. Learning to use the holes in your abilities as fuel, rather than discouragement, and continually challenging your unconscious competence in the face of a continually changing knowledge base in your sport and your own tendency towards complacency, ensures that you will also be able to grow and learn in that discomfort. You will open new doors of possibility for yourself if you can learn to override instinct, learn to change your thought process, tap into positive emotion, and develop physiological coherence.

The brain functions to regulate the body through a combination of excitatory and inhibitory activity through our Autonomic Nervous System (ANS) and hormones. Our ANS operates mainly unconsciously. The brain is involved in learning by forming new circuitry and strengthening or weakening existing circuitry, most often also unconsciously. It is also very good at selection. Whatever your experience has taught you to value, it focuses on. Whatever belief systems you have put in place that reside in your subconscious, your brain looks for evidence to support those beliefs and ignore what doesn't. It learns from what you attend to. Attention is the core mechanism that guides our awareness and experiences. *Our attention shapes our neural circuitry.* Those subconscious beliefs often filter out possibility and limit your potential. Learning to consciously expand that filter and your awareness of self-imposed limitations helps to build a new belief system based on who you really are, not who you "think" you should be.

When you learn to regulate your actions, thoughts, and emotions to create benefit rather than harm to yourself, you are changing your brain and relying on the calm of your parasympathetic nervous system to enhance your performance and your life.

In sport, the pain and discomfort that you experience while learning new things, for the most part, won't kill you but will offer two options: to hurt you or transform you. If you presume that a new skill is going to be easy, you will most likely experience anger, confusion, irritation, or even give up when it is harder than you think it should be. Learning how to deal with discomfort in a way that encourages transformation rather than avoidance overrides your primal instinct to move away from things that "hurt" or are unfamiliar, or perhaps even require us to change. Developing consciousness may trigger your existing programming to avoid that kind of awareness, because you don't even know what it is you don't know. We tend to look for answers or solutions where it is easy or familiar—not in uncomfortable, unfamiliar places where the real solutions may reside.

The Brain and Change

Our brains are both complicated and simple. They can control us and we can control them. They are simple and under our control in that, if you close your eyes right now and imagine you are somewhere other than where you actually are, your brain will believe you are there. If you tell it with imagery, visualization, and mental rehearsal that you are out on a golf course putting green practicing your short game, the same motor and sensory programs that are involved in actually doing it will be activated. Every thought will leave a physical signature that alters synapses in your brain microscopically. You can cognitively practice your skills not only mentally in your mind, but electrically and physically in your neurons.

Our brains are also complicated. The study of the brain has been called the last frontier in science. We know that there is more about the brain that we *don't* know than what we do know. The field of neuroscience is still in its infancy, which means that as we understand more about the brain and how our neurology works, there remains an incredible amount that we have not even considered yet. We have an estimated 100 billion brain cells or neurons, and each has up to 40,000 synapses or connections. A piece of brain matter the size of a grain of sand has 100,000 neurons and a billion synapses. Information can move in the brain at speeds of 260 mph (or 418 km/hr). (Queensland Brain Institute) That's some pretty impressive wiring and machinery that can control us. *How* we use that equipment, though, is really up to us, and doing the work to rewire our brains is something we can do with consciousness training to enhance our performance and our lives.

The number of thoughts you have in a day is suggested to be somewhere in the range of 6,000–50,000, with many of those thoughts being negative and repetitive. What we tell ourselves reflects not only the way we think, but also how we feel and act. In other words, our thoughts influence how we create our reality. We all know that memories can be unreliable. What and how you remember can be affected by emotions, motivations, cues, context, or even how often you remember them. Memories are more like a map than a place. They are deconstructed and stored in different areas of the brain. To be recalled, a memory has to be retrieved from several places and reconstructed. Memories are divided into two main categories: declarative facts and events, *knowing what*; and non-declarative skills and habits, *knowing how*. (Byrne, 2020) You may know both what and how to execute a skill in your sport as you move into competence, but that what and how will most likely be stored in and recalled from different areas of your brain. Learning to choose your emotions may help wire that knowing into memory so that it becomes mastery.

When you think you are in control of your life, think again. The subconscious mind controls 95 percent of how our circumstances manifest, and our beliefs shape our lives. The power of the subconscious is about a million times greater than our conscious mind (Lipton, 2016). If 95 percent of the decisions you make are done subconsciously, habitually, and you are operating on beliefs you may not even realize you have, imagine what power you can tap into by simply stepping into conscious awareness and creativity.

Our midbrain, sometimes called our mammalian brain, is where we resist change. The center in our midbrain, called the amygdala, triggers our autonomic responses to fear. Fear is a healthy response to some things. Our fight, flight, or freeze system has ensured our survival. We learn by repeated experience to fear something and respond accordingly. When you step out of your comfort zone, in any area of your life including sport, the stress alarms our amygdala. The bad news is that when you are in your midbrain resisting that discomfort or change, you cannot access your cortex or thinking brain and actually choose to change.

Very Good News

The very good news is that you can learn how to "tiptoe" around your amygdala (one of the tools discussed later), stay in your parasympathetic nervous system, and access your cortex and higher thinking. Here, you can create new "software" for the desired changes you are looking to make and establish new pathways and habits. You can teach your brain to circumvent its built-in resistance to change with consciousness. Small steps, controlled breath, positive thought, and emotion all work towards making changes from the smallest space between neurons in our brain to our biggest accomplishments in sport and life. I like to call it "neuroplastic surgery." The power in making those changes in our brains is relatively untapped potential for most of us, and in that potential, you are capable of doing much more than you could ever imagine.

It can be stressful to remain steadfast, confident, and calm in the face of what your neuroanatomy and amygdala may be telling you. Most of us react negatively and pessimistically when the amygdala is in the driver's seat. You will benefit from learning the skills to get out of that stress by acting instead of reacting, by coming into consciousness, and by finding comfort outside of your comfort zone. Those benefits will be physical, emotional, and mental. When you allow how you perform to *trans*form you rather than have you *con*form, hurt, or define you, you will be well on the way to consciousness.

When you are able to apply this psychophysiological component to your training and the choices you make, when you understand what hurts your performance and what helps, and when you learn how to let go of

> "When you allow how you *perform* to *trans*form you rather than have you *con*form, hurt, or define you, you will be well on the way to consciousness.

what hurts and strengthen what helps, you will be on the road to consciousness. Your mind will not be an unconscious ball-and-chain slowing you down, but a powerful tool under conscious control, allowing you to achieve your highest goals and your heart's desires.

6

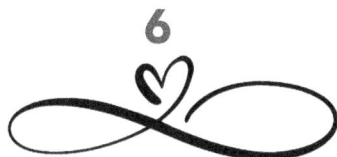

Steps to Consciousness

STEP ONE:
BE AWARE OF AND ADMIT TO
YOUR UNCONSCIOUSNESS

Connie knew how to work hard. She was accomplished in her career and in her athletics. She qualified for Kona, Hawaii, her second Ironman, and frequently won women's overall and/or her age group in triathlon and running races. She had a plan for how she would fit training into her day, every day, and kept a detailed diary of what she ate, how she felt, what her heart rate and energy level were, what workout she did, her body weight, hours of sleep, and water intake. Her awareness of her goals and her desire to get there were impressive.

Then, her world unraveled. She tore her ACL during a winter ski vacation and had to undergo surgery to have it re-attached. With no familiar routine and collection of data, who was she? What would she do? The demons that had driven her to her level of overachievement were about to rear their heads with no way for her to keep them at bay. Her underlying motivation, which was to avoid failure at all costs, began to surface.

The truth was, though, the injury was a gift. Why? Because it allowed her to bring a deeper awareness to why she was so driven to train so hard.

Her physical body had to be broken down in some way to force her to stop all activity in order for her emotional body to come into awareness, if only she would allow it. Connie was being invited into developing a healthy sense of self outside of sport and accomplishment.

Sometimes we must be knocked out of our unconsciousness. A race day that ends in perceived failure can be a disaster if we stay unconscious and struggle with only seeing what "should" have happened. The disaster can be a necessary and painful two-by-four that knocks us out of that unconsciousness, into consciousness. That's when we can learn the lessons about ourselves and see the disaster as an opportunity.

The Road Inward

If you bring forth what is within you
it will save you. If you do not bring forth
what is within you, it will destroy you.

—Gospel of Thomas

As mentioned earlier, what often directs our attention to what's going on in our consciousness is exactly the crisis that forces us to slow down or maybe even stop. We unconsciously teeter on the path of illness, injury, broken down bodies, and relationships, wondering why our performance and/or our lives are not better. Those struggles help us to realize our unconscious incompetence when we don't even know what we don't know about ourselves.

Often, living unconsciously comes from an external, rather than an internal, focus. We choose to look outside rather than inside ourselves. Maybe we mock the idea of "too much self-focus" or "looking inside." When you first start down the road of sport, the focus is often external.

There is an attachment to outcome and the opportunity to blame that outcome on someone or something else. That may serve its purpose in the beginning. Perhaps sport acted as a pacifier, a distraction, or a means to an end in the beginning; as you moved forward in your journey, a discomfort or an awareness began to surface—and it's in that discomfort and awareness that you have the opportunity to start looking less at outer achievements and more at the inner drive.

That journey inward may begin when negative consequences of training and competing start to occur. Injury, overtraining, plateauing, depression, or even lost relationships may force you to seek solutions other than another workout. You may have to begin to slow down, dig deep, and develop a consciousness of who you are and why you make the choices you do.

There may be an understanding that you are giving your power and energy away to outcome or to other people against or with whom you're competing, or that you define yourself by results and comparison rather than by a sense of who you really are apart from sports or achievement.

The truth is, developing conscious awareness isn't for cowards.

What's at Stake

When you decide to take the inner journey, you will face things you may or may not have expected to encounter. Some of those things include false beliefs and attitudes about yourself. Cognitive dissonance may be something you feel when your deeply rooted beliefs conflict with your observations of what must change. An example of that could be, you believe that training hard is good for you, but you are injured more than not. When your beliefs are inconsistent with your actions or outcomes, when you have to decide between different choices, or you are unable to receive new information that contradicts what you believe, you will feel uncomfortable at first. Your identity may feel threatened, and you may get caught trying to rationalize the dissonance to the point of feeling stressed out. The challenge is being willing to acknowledge and change them—and as you do that, I promise you the outside becomes a completely different world for you to see and to live in. How do you do that? Well, start with asking yourself some questions.

1. What are two cognitions that are not fitting together in my life?
2. How big is the conflict between them?
3. What actions can I take to reduce the dissonance?
4. Does a behavior, a belief, or my perspective need to be changed?
5. How important is it for me to reconcile the dissonance?

For many of us, deciding to examine ourselves a little deeper can be an uncomfortable process. Therefore, your instinct initially may be to move away from that discomfort and those depths. It may feel easier or better to avoid who you are than to understand yourself and, maybe for the first time, become true to who you really are. Becoming your "true self" may require the most sustained effort you have ever given.

Athletes know all about effort: how to work hard, how to push physically. Learning how to push through inner barriers can require even more effort and energy than your sport does. Not pushing through those inner barriers has costs. Walling off huge portions of our being by focusing on other portions can literally make us sick. If you are so focused on the athlete in you that you ignore, say, a wounded aspect of yourself, you may not understand why you experience symptoms of depression or other negative emotions when you are not performing or competing.

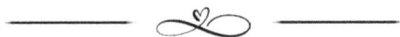

The curious paradox is that when I accept myself just as I am, then I can change.

—Carl Rogers

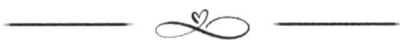

Carl Rogers, one of the fathers of humanistic psychology, speaks of "waking consciousness" from its unconscious foundations by reclaiming disowned or dark aspects of ourselves. Some of those disowned aspects may be personality traits you have been told are "bad" or "wrong," and so you have judged them harshly and kept them unconscious. When you dig a little deeper, you may find those same traits you were told were wrong can help you now in your life, or you can own them and consciously get rid of them. Rogers proposed that we all have a basic innate desire to actualize and enhance ourselves. That desire is perhaps our most basic fuel and guides the direction our lives take. Sport most certainly can be a vehicle to do just that if we become conscious of using it to fulfill that basic need of *guiding* our lives rather than *being* our whole lives.

When you are out of contact with your own needs, feelings, emotions, frustrations, and longings, you may be oblivious to who you actually are. Your life may have become a reflection of your "unreal" self, of a role you have merely adopted that you think you are supposed to be playing. You become disconnected from your inner experience by focusing on the outer. If you are more concerned about the results of your race season than you are about how much joy you experienced during that season, you may be looking in the wrong direction.

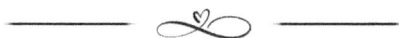

No sooner do we think that we have
assembled a comfortable life than we find
a piece of ourselves with no place to fit in.

—Gail Sheehy

Where do I Begin?

We are all coming from different places in our journeys. There is no straight line or simple formula to be a better athlete or more aware person. The very first step can be an admission that sport has a power over you and the consequences have become too much. You can simply start where you are and move forward to a deeper place and add to your existing state of being. No matter where your starting point is, you can develop new tools to step into your own power and get to where it is you want to go. You may overcome fear, get faster, challenge an existing attitude about your life or your training, and start to understand why it is you feel the need to measure yourself against others.

The perceived disaster of the ACL tear that Connie experienced was her wake-up call to the starting line of becoming conscious. While her body healed, she took time to reflect on the uncomfortable questions she had never asked herself: Why did she train so hard, and what was she looking for? Where was she in cognitive dissonance? The why and the what came into greater focus and alignment when she allowed herself to be in the discomfort of having to sit still. She discovered in that stillness what she had been running from and why she was doing the running. Looking inside herself helped her make changes that nothing outside of herself could. When she returned to racing, she had found a sense of peace and satisfaction she had never known before. She spent more time reflecting on what she learned about herself training and racing rather than recording data and accumulating medals.

If you have an open attitude, a thirst to learn more about yourself, and a desire to know how who you are now is inhibiting you from becoming who you choose to be, you will be able to move out of your unconscious state.

You may recognize that you have never even thought about some of the things talked about in this book. You may have not wanted to look at why you work so hard to be good at your sport even when there is diminishing return on your effort, or you may have been looking in the wrong places to improve your performance. You may feel stuck but not know how to get out of the rut you are in. There may be a high external focus with no awareness of the inner motivation to excel. You may have spent all your time pushing towards your goals out of fear instead of being pulled towards them out of love, joy, and passion. Negative emotions like fear are always about resistance, while positive emotions like joy are about allowing or resonance. Learning to live in the positive and being drawn towards your goals is most certainly worth practicing.

Over the years, I have found that awareness brings success in whatever you are doing. Unconscious forces that push you can be identified and dealt with only when you become aware of them. You must challenge yourself, find out what you are *not* dealing with, where you may not be authentic in your words and actions, and start aligning your actions with who you are as your consciousness expands. A way to start this process is to simply become an observer of your thoughts and feelings. Consciousness requires owning your emotions, thoughts, and actions without judgment or repression. Then you can allow them to lead you to a greater sense of self. Be in as much of a state of mindfulness as you can possibly be. It can negate the need to "run away from ourselves."

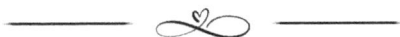

―――――――― ❧ ――――――――

All human beings should try to learn before they die
what they are running from, and to, and why.

—James Thurber

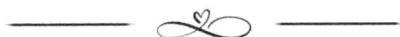

―――――――― ❧ ――――――――

STEP TWO:
PRACTICE WITH BEGINNER'S MIND

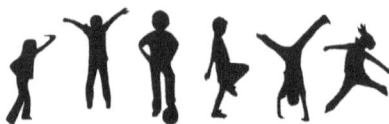

In the beginner's mind, there are many possibilities;
in the expert's mind, there are few.

—Shunryu Suzuki

One of my favorite questions is, "When was the last time you did something for the first time?"

As we get older, we tend to do the things we know how to do. We may resist new things, feeling like we are not good at something for fear of being judged by others or even by ourselves. We don't want to look silly when we fail or for people to laugh at us when we can't do something they can. Children don't worry about such things. They delight in attempting things they cannot do and "failing." Watching a toddler learning how to walk is quite impressive in their obliviousness to what we would call failure. They fall, get back up, fall again, get back up again until they learn how to stand steady on their own two little feet. When was the last time you learned something with such determination and such little obvious success?

> When was the
> last time you did
> something for the
> first time?

Sue had competed at the Olympic level in flatwater kayaking and cross-country skiing. She was an exceptional athlete. As she approached her 60s, she decided that she needed to start working on her flexibility in order to extend her life in sport. Her first yoga class was eye-opening. She was unable to do most of what the instructor asked of her and was sweating in the first five minutes on the mat. She was delighted. She had found something new and fun that challenged her, and knew that with some practice and patience, she would most certainly get better. That hour of yoga had her laughing more than she could remember in the past year. That same curious and open mind that got her to the Olympic Games was there on that yoga mat, ready to explore and learn.

The beginner or childlike mind has nothing to resist, so the natural progression of awareness of error, practice of correction, and then progress is completely natural and allows for quick learning. There is a pacing with small steps, not leaps and bounds like an experienced athlete might expect. A beginner's mind is not clogged with a history of data, results, and beliefs that stops them from being a better athlete and person. Beginners don't have built-up egos that stop them from learning new things at which they might not yet be proficient. They are always in a learning mode—paying close attention, not checking out because they think they already know something. They practice with ease and patience, not effort and force. They understand their body will warn them of potential illness or injury and are more likely to listen to that warning rather than have to suffer the consequences of ignoring it. A novice mind will patiently take a break, while those with experience, more often than not, give it one last push.

What flows through your mind sculpts your brain. With an open mind, you have the ability to form new circuits and strengthen or weaken existing ones. In learning to observe that flow and consciously choose positive thoughts, images, and emotions, you can change your brain for the better. Regulating words, thoughts, and emotions to create benefit rather than harm, to enhance performance rather than inhibit, is a practice you can become exceptional at if you are open to it.

Our "mind" can be considered as information the nervous system moves, just like our heart moves blood through our body. Most of the information flowing through our brains and nervous system is outside our awareness. If you make a conscious decision to look at what passes through your mind, and the rhythm your heart is beating in, you can decide what helps you as an athlete. Then you can learn to strengthen what helps and let go of what doesn't. You may feel very much like a beginner at first, learning to observe your thoughts and emotions—and while in that conscious incompetence, you may become frustrated when you are not good at it and don't see immediate improvement. Stay open and allow your beginner's mind to take you to new heights of awareness and performance.

With an expanded consciousness and awareness, there can be much more opportunity to learn and to grow. In *The Warrior Athlete,* Dan Millman tells us that learning is a response to a demand to grow, and most certainly will involve error (Millman, 1979). In order to correct an error, you must bring awareness to it. That awareness can include knowledge, cognizance, being vigilant and mindful of sensory feedback, mental clarity, and emotional intuition. It is easy to focus on what we do well; it is much harder to be aware of and focus on what we don't do so well. Whether you are brand new to a sport or have mastered skills necessary to compete at high levels, beginner 's mind allows growth towards levels of skill you may not even know are possible or necessary.

I tell most of my athletes that in order to help them get to the next level of their ability and performance, I will more than likely have them focus on things they are not aware of, open to, or good at yet. They will also have to be open to changing what they think they already know. It can be a seemingly disillusioning process, requiring you to check your ego at first, and most likely, you will get worse before you get better. In the long run, though, working on the things you don't do well by bringing awareness to them will make you a better athlete. Humility and patience can be difficult and rare amongst athletes, but to me as a coach, it represents a willingness to learn and to grow. Looking inside ourselves as an opportunity to become better athletes is a way to bring positivity to what we often perceive as negative, a way to bring consciousness to unconsciousness.

Awareness can move beyond the physical body; it can mean being open to a deeper understanding of what is going on and why. Even when you're working on and mastering the physical skills, you can start to look inside and bring your awareness to a natural rhythm, an understanding, a wisdom and intuitiveness that allows you to not just be a better athlete, but a more mindful person. If you are learning to change a skill you have practiced for many years, you may notice that you get frustrated and actually get worse before you get better. Being aware of your response and laughing at yourself instead of getting more frustrated will decrease your resistance to the change and increase your awareness of how learning a new skill is not just a physical process.

The brain and its thought process focus less energy on the body and bring more awareness to the depths of who you are and why you do the things you do. Sometimes, something you were not even aware of comes into focus or becomes clear as you shift your awareness to what is really going on in and around you. Beginner's mind is understanding and recognizing that our incredible, intellectual, thinking minds not only helped us achieve success in many ways, but also distorted and blocked things from our view that have the potential to help us exceed our existing or perceived limits. If we consciously set aside our filters, open our minds to possibilities, look for new ways to do old things on purpose and perhaps even for the fun of it—if we use "I don't know" as a strategy even when we think we do "know," then secrets previously unavailable to us become known. Why? Because we have cleared the mind of thought and remained wide open, thus allowing new insights and answers to arise.

When life is scary and difficult, we tend to look for answers and solutions in the easy or familiar places, not in the hard or uncomfortable ones where real solutions may lie. Stepping out of ego and into essence is something we can all practice in sport and in life. Being cautious and curious as you explore outside your current limits rather than fearful and doubtful in your safe box may open up doors to possibilities previously limited by our old beliefs and reactive nervous system. Who knows how far you can go with your performance when you can listen and practice new things, even when you are skeptical; when you are open to possibility rather than stuck in impossibility, even if you "think" it can't be done.

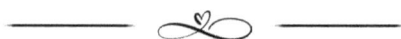

———————— ❦ ————————

Curiosity will conquer fear
even more than bravery will.

—James Stephens

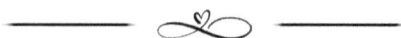

———————— ❦ ————————

STEP THREE:
TAKE INVENTORY OF YOUR SELF

*How few there are who have courage
enough to own their faults, or resolution
enough to mend them.*

—Benjamin Franklin

The way to improve your life consciously is by honestly and willingly evaluating what kind of person you really are and then deciding who you really want to be. For many of us, this can be a scary and difficult thing to do. It's easy to look at other people and see the changes you think they may need to make in their lives, but it's much harder to look at ourselves. We may not even realize that we have limiting beliefs and biases, let alone know how to let go of them. Being biased doesn't help us grow, it just hides the beliefs we are resistant to change or acknowledge. Understand this: it is through the realization of our false beliefs and imperfections that is the way to great potential. The more things you are willing to look at and change in yourself, the more opportunity you will have to grow as a conscious athlete and human being.

One of my favorite tools for self-analysis is the Johari Window, created in 1955 by Joseph Luft and Harry Ingham (Luft and Ingham, 1969). It is a simple and useful model for understanding and practicing self-awareness and personal development. There are basically four quadrants to the model:

Quadrant One is open. This is where aspects of yourself are known to you and to others. For example, John knows he is a hard worker and everyone on his team knows he is also. This is the quadrant you want to enlarge as you expand your consciousness. You will want to strengthen these qualities and put them to good use.

Johari Window model

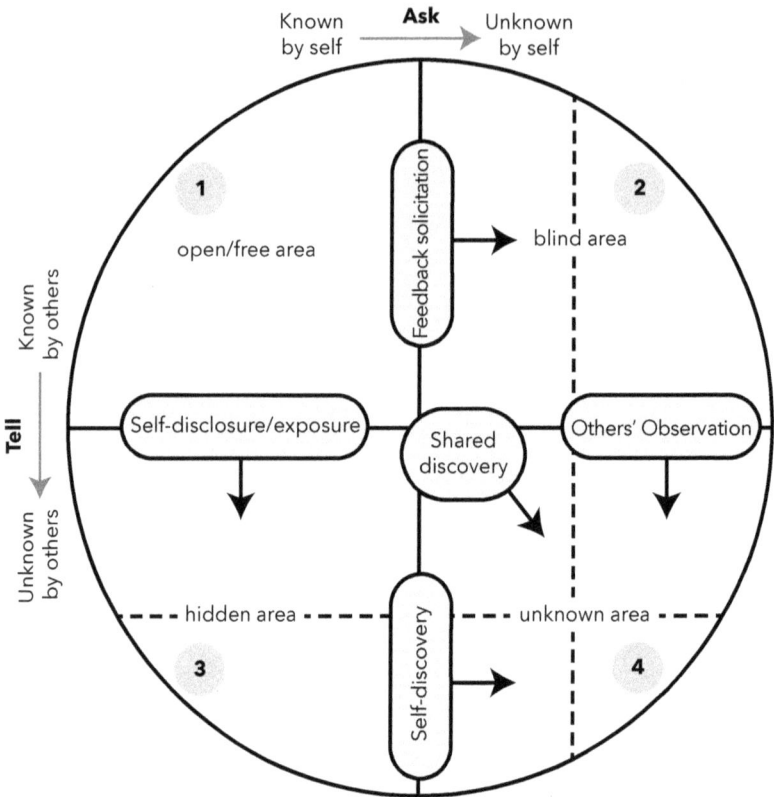

In Quadrant Three, there are aspects of yourself that you are aware of, but hide from others. John thinks he is not a "talented" athlete and is afraid of making mistakes in games. His teammates have no idea of his fear. You are conscious of something that you think is "bad" or a perceived weakness and believe it may result in alienation from others. Learning to overcome weaknesses takes courage, awareness, and patience.

Quadrant Two is a blind spot. You are ignorant of yourself and your issues, but others see them. Here is where you can solicit feedback from people you trust to tell you the truth. John's teammates know he is too hard on himself and could learn to enjoy playing more. You are unconscious of things that may be limiting your potential. Becoming more introspective and opening up to the insight of others may be scary at first, but laughable when you eventually own the resistance you had.

Quadrant Four is completely unknown to you and to others. This is where there may lay some deep-rooted fears along with some deeply buried talents. The big challenge is to realize what is buried in that fear. Often, it takes adversity for that to happen. Accepting the obvious challenges in life, or even facing the unimaginable ones, help us to realize those hidden qualities and fears. If you did not have opportunity, training, encouragement, or confidence to display some hidden ability, you may find something here in the unknown that changes your game and your life. John's team was down by two goals in the last few minutes of their championship game. Much to John's surprise, the coach put him on the field and told the other players to feed him the ball and for him to shoot as many times as he possibly could in the remaining time. John had never felt so much pressure in his life. He was unaware of the ability he had inside that would be revealed in those last few minutes and under that pressure. He scored three goals in record time and won the game for his team.

Studying and having a deep knowledge of your sport is very important in order for you to perform at high levels. The study of self is really the highest form of study in existence that there is. It requires a commitment to change rather than maintaining the status quo. Understanding your sport and yourself means not only looking at skills and physiology, but also knowing your own mind and emotions. When you own, realize, and understand how you feel and why you do the things you do, you live a much more purposeful and aligned life. The stirrings of our inner being may fuel an exterior world that makes more sense.

Figuring out who you are is not for the faint of heart. It is an ongoing process that might take months, even years, and there is no one way to do it. Practiced continually, though, it is the solution to personal growth and internal advancement. Asking for feedback from people we trust is a way to start opening the window to your real self. If you encourage feedback from trusted individuals about what they see in you, without your resistance to their feedback, you bring to light parts of yourself you can own and parts you may want to discard.

Self-knowledge holds the keys and teaches us the techniques to develop our consciousness and then use it in our lives. Knowing yourself helps you make sense of your life and how you live it and will help you understand how you can show up better as an athlete.

Self-analysis requires you to look at your beliefs, thoughts, and behaviors and often to ask for help in discovering what you are missing or may even be denying. In your blind spot, there is an ignorance of yourself that would benefit you to bring into awareness. Many of us do not see the potential we have or the limitations we have unconsciously put on ourselves.

I have found that the things people don't want to hear are most often the things they need to hear. When my athletes push back on my observations of them or are sensitive to hearing things they don't realize about themselves, I know I have hit a spot that they don't want to own. Risking exposure is not easy. Opening our eyes to the truth of ourselves can be hard. The good news is that the less blind we are to ourselves, the more authentic we can become, and operate from a place of consciousness rather than out of habit or old belief systems.

Each and every one of us has a potential power hidden deeply inside. My job has been to help my athletes find and own that power. When faced with unexpected adversity, all of the athletes I have ever coached were grateful for the lessons that adversity had to offer them. It may not have happened in the immediate aftermath of the adversity, but eventually they opened themselves up to what they were supposed to learn. We often don't tap into our real power because we are more attached to outcome and satisfaction than we are to the lessons we can learn, despite the outcome. We are looking for something in return like appreciation, money, or status. Maybe we love the respect we get from being the top athlete in our field. To realize our true potential, however, we must take a hard look at the inside of ourselves without being attached to those outer sources or rewards.

In the dark unknown areas of the subconscious mind, there are behaviors, attitudes, capabilities, and aptitudes that can be positive and useful once revealed. Or there can be aspects of your personality influencing your behavior in a negative way that limits you. You may be pleasantly surprised when an unexpected challenge calls for deeply buried abilities to rise to the surface. Old beliefs you have about your life and yourself may have a choke hold on you and limit your performance, your relationships, and other important areas of your world.

Even the fastest people on the planet are always looking to get faster. They eventually must do something different.

"My coach says I don't need to stretch."

"I always eat steak the night before I race."

"Lifting weights is a waste of time."

"Suck it up. We have all been injured. It's no excuse to stop training."

We all tend to search for, select, recall, and interpret information that confirms our beliefs, even in the face of information that contradicts it. When we have an emotional charge associated with our belief, we stay even more entrenched, despite evidence to the contrary of what we believe. Being open to changing those biases opens us up to possibilities we never imagined.

What passes through our minds is often not true; it is only what we believe to be true. Focusing on one point of view or possibility while ignoring or dismissing alternatives can lead to poor decisions and poor performance.

Beliefs run in your subconscious mind. They are formed through the experiences you have in life and the thoughts you have rendered as to what is the absolute truth about your world. Beliefs are the "blueprints" of your life, the plans you lay down in your youth with the thoughts you render as truth about your life and your world.

Imagine this scenario:

As a small child, your parents enrolled you in swim lessons. Your first day there, all suited up in your new bathing suit, goggles, and cap, the instructor decided to have the class jump in the deep end of the pool. One child protested that they didn't want to do that, so the instructor promptly picked that child up, walked them over to the edge of the pool, and dropped them into the water. You watched in horror, thinking that you were the next to be thrown in. A belief was formed in that experience that swimming in deep water was a very scary thing to do and instructors were definitely *not* to be trusted.

Now, as an adult, you find yourself not wanting to be around pools or in water over your head. You know that you could learn how to swim with a better instructor, but subconsciously, every time you think about taking a class, you get uncomfortable and opt not to. This is because you didn't take the time to change that belief, and it stayed embedded in your subconscious mind, perhaps limiting your desire to take up the sport of triathlon that you recently have become really interested in.

You must start with the desire to make changes to improve your performance. There must be a burning desire for constant self-improvement to occur. We get comfortable in our old ways and resist change. Moving out of those comfort zones can be difficult. Even if we are unhappy there, it is still familiar and comfortable. Often, we choose to run back to safe, old ways rather than move forward in unfamiliar ways that we are not necessarily good at yet.

You must then identify what you desire to change. You can only change something when you identify it. Once you know the belief that is holding you back, you have the opportunity to give it a new, positive meaning. You may notice yourself saying or thinking negative statements that reinforce your false belief about the water and instructor when you were a child:

> "I can't swim."
> "I don't like the water."
> "Instructors are mean."

Those statements are caused by the chokehold the limiting belief has on you. Learning to carefully identify your beliefs can help you understand why you may be choosing those negative, limiting words. When you have limiting or negative thoughts and belief systems, more often than not, you learned them in your youth or childhood. Those negative thoughts and beliefs can result in depression, low self-esteem, self-doubt and judgment, blaming others, thinking you are not good enough, and procrastination.

Even the most successful people experience fear and self-doubt and unconsciously hold limiting beliefs. So many elite athletes in the world have painfully revealed their stories of how they suffered with depression, eating disorders, and lack of self-esteem, and they cannot really enjoy what they have achieved, even when it is a scholarship at a Division I school or an Olympic gold medal. Joyce M. Roche, author of *The Empress Has No Clothes: Conquering Self-Doubt to Embrace Success*, puts it this way:

> Imposter syndrome is the fear and self-doubt that causes people to question their abilities —even in the face of success—and to constantly search for external validation. Simply put, it makes it difficult to recognize and celebrate one's strengths and accomplishments. They don't believe that who they are is enough or deserving, so they try to prove it with accomplishment. (Roche, 2013)

I certainly came face to face with my own limiting beliefs while exploring my unconsciousness over the years. The core beliefs of feeling unworthy of love and not being enough resulted in constant fear and doubt. The imposter I felt like tried to disprove those beliefs with accomplishment. I had spent most of my time and energy trying to be who I thought people wanted me to be and prove myself to be worthy and "enough" in the realm of sport. There was no medal big enough to ever do that. The truth was, false beliefs rooted in childhood had to be released in order for me to become the genuine star of my life. When I learned that I held the belief of not being in control of my life, it made sense that I had allowed other people to guide it. And in feeling out of control, the need to hold on for dear life was the compensation pattern and belief that I developed. Neither served me, but certainly served my old and unhealthy belief system. Releasing those beliefs required a level of trust in myself and care of myself that I had never practiced before. It felt like I was going into battle against a voice in my head that I had thought for years was my own. Undoing that unconscious programming has been a practice. I am now in the driver's seat of my life and have learned to let go of what I thought I had to hold on to for dear life. The love of my life has become my life.

Clara Hughes is a six-time Olympic medalist in cycling and speed skating. She is the only athlete in history to win multiple medals in both the Summer and Winter Olympic Games. She carried the flag for her home country of Canada in the 2010 Vancouver Winter Olympics where their Olympic team had a historic medal-winning games. Her athletic achievements rival any athlete on the planet. But there is more to Clara than her athletic ability: she was brave enough to share the story of her struggle with depression in the midst of the Olympic medal glory. Looking back, she saw that her depression started in the mid-1990s while she was training as an Olympic cyclist. "No matter what I won, I still had this void and darkness and oftentimes feelings of self-loathing and worthlessness inside," she said.

She documented the years of her struggle and the journey to where she is now in her life in her book, *Open Heart, Open Mind*. She stands on the platform of her years of struggle as an athlete and Olympian, now as a humanitarian and motivator making a difference in the lives of many people who suffer from mental health issues.

There are many similar stories of athletes—elite, Olympic, professional, amateur, weekend warriors—carrying the same beliefs and struggling with the same demons. The good news is you can learn how to release yourself from those demons and reclaim your potential. When you free yourself from limiting beliefs, you become unlimited in your potential. You can experience greater control in your life, have clarity in the decisions you make, find happiness and confidence, experience more opportunity and synchronicity, and gain greater ability to focus on what matters to you in life.

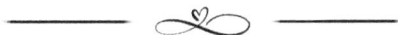

———— ❧ ————

Whatever we plan in our subconscious mind and nourish with repetition and emotion will one day become a reality.

—Earl Nightingale

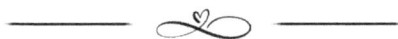

———— ❧ ————

Understanding that you are the one who laid down the blueprints of your life means you can also change those blueprints. You can come to understand that you are not your beliefs—you simply created them to deal with the reality you experienced during your life. We all attribute meaning to what we experience and hold that meaning in our minds. That meaning you gave to your experience is what causes you to feel the way you do. Acknowledging that it was you who chose what meaning to give your experiences and created the blueprints of your beliefs will most certainly make it easier for you to change them.

Our true selves often lay buried under fears and learned behavior. That true self exists whether we can excavate it or not. When we recognize our power, our luminosity, and our divinity, we cannot help but live authentic lives of appreciation, potential, fulfillment, and grace.

That little child who watched the instructor throw another young student into the deep end of the water could have interpreted the whole situation differently. They could have thought that it was a playful way to start the class, or that the instructor was having a bad day. When you are young, you don't have the ability to understand what is going through adult minds, so you decide on your own that it is about you.

You created a story that made sense to your childlike mind to explain behavior you didn't understand, and so began the laying down of a blueprint of you, by you, attributing meaning to an event that had none until you decided what it was. The meaning you gave to that event, that you could not learn how to swim, made you feel the way you do as an adult, triggered by fear around water.

When you take your inventory, you realize that your limitations and beliefs were self-imposed and can be changed. You step into the power and possibility of who you really are, not who you were told or falsely believed you were.

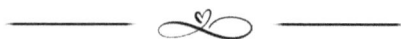

What we can or cannot do, what we consider
possible or impossible, is rarely a function
of our true capability. It is more likely a function
of our beliefs about who we are.

—Tony Robbins

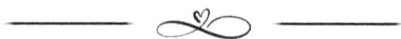

STEP FOUR:
DEDICATED, DELIBERATE PRACTICE
WITH INTENTIONAL EXCELLENCE

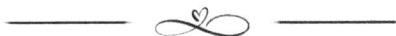

Whatever we hope to do with ease, we must first learn to do with diligence.

—Samuel Johnson

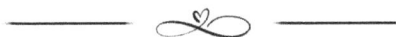

Excellence is not random. It is developed by design. The best performers are great at observing themselves, focusing intently on what they are doing, and monitoring what is happening in their minds. They are aware and can analyze their own learning and thinking processes. Learning how to have knowledge about your own knowledge, to think about your own thinking, and having awareness and understanding of your own thought and emotional processes takes you to new levels. This intentional higher order thinking and feeling enables analysis, control, and understanding of one's cognitive processes, especially when engaged in learning.

The older we get and the more years we spend on the playing field, the more we want to keep doing what we are good at and what we know how to do. We don't become excellent or masterful at something without intention. There is always room for improvement when you are able to see what you could do better. Staying in your comfort zone is not going to lead to improvement. Moving into discomfort and stretching yourself and your abilities is where changes happen. Conscious performers learn to compare themselves to something that stretches them just beyond their current limits, and they take responsibility for the process in getting there. You don't often hear elites complaining about the cold weather conditions or equipment malfunctions to explain away a less-than-exceptional performance.

Intentional excellence instead of intentional (or perhaps unintentional) mediocrity can move you towards success instead of failure in most of your life. When you act with intentional excellence, you know how to turn a previously perceived negative into a positive with swift, conscious, deliberate action. You move towards success even when you fail. When you act with mediocrity, you become negative when you see that same perceived negative in your performance and do nothing but move into a reactive, negative emotion. You move towards failure instead of success. That thin line between success and failure can be crossed quickly with intention and emotion. Excellence moves towards success, and mediocrity moves towards failure. There is no losing, only learning and winning.

Often the gains we make in sport come from the least expected places. Learning to train smarter rather than harder often takes a series of setbacks. If you want to swim faster, you swim faster, right? Well, you do until there is a point of diminishing returns. Albert Einstein said that man's greatest invention was compound interest. You might think of money when you hear that, a way to make money work for you without having to work for it. That same principle can apply to speed gains without having to work harder.

To swim faster, you want to maximize forward speed. Speed is limited by drag, turns, and technique. Speed is enhanced by power, turns, and technique. It's easier to reduce drag than it is to increase power. Doubling speed quadruples drag (which doesn't seem very fair to me), but improving your body roll and alignment and better swimsuit technology will compound your speed without you having to work any harder.

You can achieve more power and efficiency with a more stable, mobile, and stronger body. A weak core, tight shoulders, and no functional strength result in more thrashing and energy wasted. The result of that thrashing with a weak, unstable, tight body will most likely be injury rather than power or progress. All the speed you think you "should" be getting with that extra thrashing effort is simply wasted with the inefficient application of power and technique. In this scenario, the energy is left at the bottom of the pool, rather than moving you forward faster—you have spent energy, but ultimately wasted it.

I don't know about you, but I certainly don't want to spend money or energy with no return. I would rather have both provide gains with the least, the smartest, and the most conscious effort on my part.

You may not aspire to be elite, but you may want to be better at your sport. Applying the principles of the elite to your practice and desire to improve, you will find a sense of accomplishment and joy.

There is a story from the Tour De France about gains in performance coming from something as simple as bedding and pillows. Dave Brailsford, the general manager and performance director of Team Sky, Great Britain's professional cycling team, coined the term "aggregation of marginal gains." He knew that it wasn't just hard work that won the Tour. He knew that when there was a small improvement in every area related to cycling, then all those small improvements combined would bring big gains to performance. He called it the one percent margin for improvement. One of the marginal differences he knew he could make was to provide each of his riders with a sleep environment suited specifically to their bodies and preferences, including their bedding and pillows. The right pillow won't win you the tour, but it can certainly make sure that you don't lose because you are not rested enough for those 21 days of incredible effort.

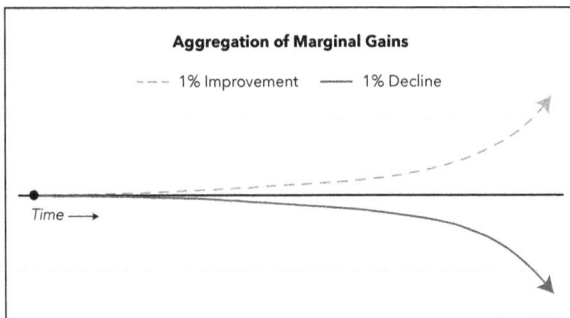

Aggregation of Marginal Gains

--- 1% Improvement   —— 1% Decline

Time ⟶

In the beginning, Brailsford knew that there was basically no difference between making a choice that is one percent better or one percent worse. Initially, you won't see the consequences or gains of that one percent choice. As time goes on, these small improvements or declines compound (just like Einstein tells us), and you suddenly find a very big difference between making the marginally better decision on a daily basis than the marginally worse. This is why small choices don't make much of a difference at the time, but do add up over the long term. Excellence doesn't happen overnight. It happens each and every day in subtle and sometimes undetectable ways, and suddenly, what was thought to be impossible becomes possible.

Success is a few simple disciplines, practiced every day; while failure is simply a few errors in judgment, repeated every day.

—Jim Rohn

One of my favorite moments in coaching is when an athlete does something they never thought or believed they could do, and in that moment, look at me with wide eyes and a big smile, sometimes even a victorious fist pump, astonished and thrilled at their accomplishment. Laurie was one of my athletes who worked for two years to get her first pull-up at age 65. When she started, she could barely hold her own weight to hang on the bar. The arm's length distance to lift herself up to that bar seemed more like 100 miles. I promised her she would get her first pull-up if she trusted that even when she didn't think she was making progress, she was. She was committed to her goal and trusted my guidance. Grip strength, shoulder shrugs, hollow body ab work, rowing, cable pulls, along with visualization and positive thoughts and statements were just some of the things she did to chip away at marginal gains to success. You would have thought she won a gold medal when she accomplished that first pull-up. It was such a privilege and joy to share that moment with her. She laughed when I said to her afterwards, "Now you really know what I told you is true. Anything you set your mind and heart to is possible."

Athletes who are productive and successful practice the things that are important on a consistent basis. Every day, they do what needs to be done in a logical, progressive, committed way. They focus on continual practice, not about the performance or outcome. You can't predict when your body is going to set a new personal record, but having a structured, dedicated, intentional practice can make sure that you're working when it does. It's about practicing your skills, not performing at a certain level. It's not the game or the event, but the practice. Accomplishments on a consistent basis require a schedule to follow, not a deadline to race toward. Successful athletes know that the journey is what counts, after all, not the destination.

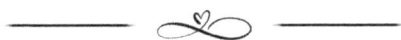

It's good to have an end to journey toward,
but in the end, it is the journey that matters.

—Ursula K. Le Guin

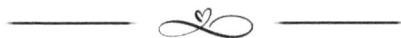

A dedicated practice with intentional excellence might include new skills: looking inward, breathing, pivoting, neurofeedback, anxiety management, meditation, affirmation, reframing, visualization, conscious thought and emotion, or measuring success using a new standard. The new skills and standards require patience and a period of resistance and unfamiliarity. Learning how to change and control what "passes through your mind and heart" is most certainly a task most of us have not considered as athletes. To be deliberate and dedicated to that will most certainly change your life as an athlete and as a person. With intentional excellence, the impossible may become possible.

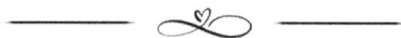

It takes consistent, repetitive, intentional
intention to become the best at what we can do.

—Dr. J. Dispenza

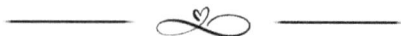

STEP FIVE:
INTENTIONAL GENERATION OF COHERENCE

*By learning to control the heart,
we can reclaim control of our emotions.*

—David Servan-Schreiber

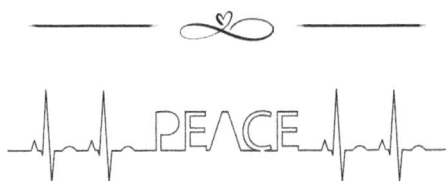

The definition of coherence is rooted in a Latin word meaning "stick together." It brings to mind a logical and orderly consistent relationship between parts.

Neurofeedback is a cutting-edge technology that is being used to enhance athletic performance. From the University of Utah, Dr. D. Corydon Hammond tells us that "neurofeedback (EEG biofeedback) holds potential for retraining brainwave activity to enhance optimal performance in athletes in various sports." (Hammond, 2011) "Neurofeedback has the potential to retrain the brain waves' activities to improve performance and attention of athletes in various sports disciplines. It is suggested to sport psychologists that use these methods for improving attention and performance." (Fallah, 2018) Improving concentration, focus, cognitive function, and emotional control are brain changing and performance enhancing techniques. By looking at your brain waves, you can teach your mind to be active in the right areas to help you perform better. Imagine being able to stop mental chatter, sharpen your focus, and keep your anxiety at a level that enhances your performance rather than inhibits it? Learning how to use the communication from your heart to your brain and body systems is a way to do just that.

In a concise view of our brain and mind, you have two: a neuro*logical* brain and neuro*emotional* brain. The way you perceive information and form thoughts will be through one of those brains. Your logical brain will deal with facts or truths about an event to create a plan of action as a result of your "logical thinking." Your emotional brain will deal with feelings or perceptions about that event to create a plan of action as a result of your "emotional feeling." Emotions will always trump logic. The two brains are always involved in the perception of your world. Thought is inherently an emotional process. Learning to intentionally generate an emotion that creates a plan to enhance your performance rather than sabotage it is something you can practice and learn to consciously do.

Altering your physiological, emotional, and cognitive state to a more positive frame and orderly relationship (coherence), will enhance your performance. What eventually separates elite athletes from the rest of us comes down to their ability to manage their emotional state under the stress of competition. They don't have less stress than you do, but they are better equipped to handle it and not have it impact their performance negatively. They have developed their awareness to levels that allow them to be focused and in control of their thoughts, emotions, and physiology and, as a result, their performance. If you have not heard of psychophysiological coherence and heart rate variability, it's time you were introduced to this skill you have waiting inside you to tap into.

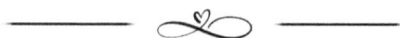

---

*Thinking is also about feeling and it is actually
neurobiologically impossible to have any
meaningful and complex thought without
some kind of emotional content.*

—Mary-Helen Immordino-Yang, Ed.D.

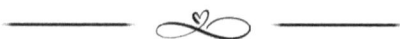

Learning to combine your physical, mental, and emotional training will give you a true competitive advantage and you will be able to find that place we call "the zone" with more consistency. The zone could be considered a "coherent physiological state" that you access with your emotions and perceptions, enabling you to experience a positive domino effect in your performance: greater clarity in thinking and decision-making; greater achievement from your body; greater resilience after adversity.

Performance = Potential – Interference
(Gallowey, 1997)

The math tells us that to increase performance and tap into your potential, you must minimize interference. If you react to disruption, distraction, or outcome negatively, you will diminish performance. Learning to control your reaction to things you cannot control will help you tap into your potential. How many times have you seen athletes throw their tennis racket, golf club, lacrosse stick or baseball bat when their game is not going as planned? The negative emotion that they display unleashes all kinds of interference in their bodies. There are thousands of biochemical changes that overload the nervous system and, as a result, the physical potential the athlete worked so hard to develop is not accessible mentally. Performance is compromised and the long-term effects of chronic reactiveness will reduce performance, resiliency, and will eventually take you out of the game. Athletes who train consciously—physically, mentally, and emotionally—will have an advantage over their competitors and will be better equipped to consistently find their potential and peak performance zone.

There is no getting away from stress, but there are ways of reducing our resistance and reaction to it. In order to compete at higher levels, you not only have to improve your performance and skills, you have to improve your ability to deal with the increased stress. Going from the starting line of a local 5K to the starting line of your state championships is still the same starting line, but your perception of the "stress" on that starting line is higher at the one you deem more important. Your talent, along with your temperament, your perception of challenge or pressure, and the ability to be calm, positive, and confident rather than anxious, negative, and fearful are all factors that will affect your performance positively or negatively depending on how you deal with that increased stress.

HeartMath® Institute's science and research shows how learning to be in coherence helps change habitual emotional patterns that are a major source of stress. Installing new emotional patterns enhances and supports performance, health, and wellbeing. Coherence is a highly efficient physiological state where the cardiovascular, nervous, hormonal, and immune systems are balanced, in sync, and work efficiently and harmoniously with energetic coordination. The way into this state of coherence is through your heart and your emotions. You may have experienced "the zone" in your athletic career and know how profound it is to be there. We have a higher consciousness where life and experiences can be processed from another level of intelligence. It is a state of heart-brain synchronization where higher motor faculties and intuition equals a flow, a coordination, a way to exceed perceived limits in a magical and mystical state of *deliberately* altered consciousness.

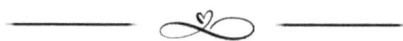

Knowing how you actually want to feel is the most potent form of clarity that you can have. Generating those feelings is the most powerfully creative thing you can do with your life.

—Danielle LaPorte

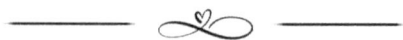

You may think of your heart as just a muscle and a pump that responds to the orders given to it by the body and the brain. Knowing our heart rate, how it responds to effort or load, and how quickly it recovers is part of most training programs. Fitness may be measured by improvements in your cardiac function. Heart rate monitors are one of the top selling training devices on the market. We now know the heart is much more—much smarter, more intuitive—than just how fast it is beating.

Historically, the heart has been regarded as a source of wisdom, intuition, and emotion. Research over the past few decades has shown that those associations are not just metaphorical. We now know the heart is a hormonal gland that makes and secretes hormones and neurotransmitters that affect brain and body function. The emerging science of neuro-cardiology has discovered that the heart has its own nervous system with over 40,000 neurons that can sense and process information, make decisions, and even demonstrate learning and memory. It has been referred to as our second or little brain. Our hearts actually talk more to our brains than our brains talk to our hearts, and not just about processing emotions. Heart signals affect higher cognitive faculties including memory, problem solving, attention, and perception. (Science of the Heart Volume 2, 2015).

Your heart rate variability (HRV), simply put, is the beat-to-beat changes in heart rate or its natural fluctuations. Short-term beat-to-beat changes are generated and amplified by the interaction or flow of neural signals between the heart and the brain. HRV is a measure of neuro-cardiac function that reflects heart-brain interactions and autonomic nervous system dynamics, along with the ability to adapt to stress or living situations. It is an indicator of health and fitness and a marker of resilience and behavioral flexibility. It can also be looked at as a marker of biological aging and reflects our stress levels and emotional state.

If you graphed those small beat-to-beat changes, you would see a pattern or a rhythm that is directly related to emotional dynamics and physiological synchronization. Breath, exercise, thoughts, and especially emotions all affect the heart's changing rhythm. When you are in a negative emotion, like anger, anxiety, or frustration, you have an irregular and erratic wave that looks like a series of jagged and uneven peaks—an incoherent heart rhythm pattern. The two branches of the ANS are out of balance and you are in cortical inhibition, which can limit everything from how you move to how you perceive what is happening around you. Your adrenals dump the stress hormones adrenaline and cortisol into your body, brain function is inhibited, and decision making is impaired: not something you want happening in the last quarter of your basketball game when you are down by three points. You can think of it like driving a car with one foot on the brake (your parasympathetic nervous system: PNS) and the other on the accelerator (your sympathetic nervous system: SNS) at the same time, creating a jerky, inefficient ride. Just as that would be bad for your car, it is also bad for your body to operate in inefficiency, depleting energy and putting extra wear and tear on our body systems.

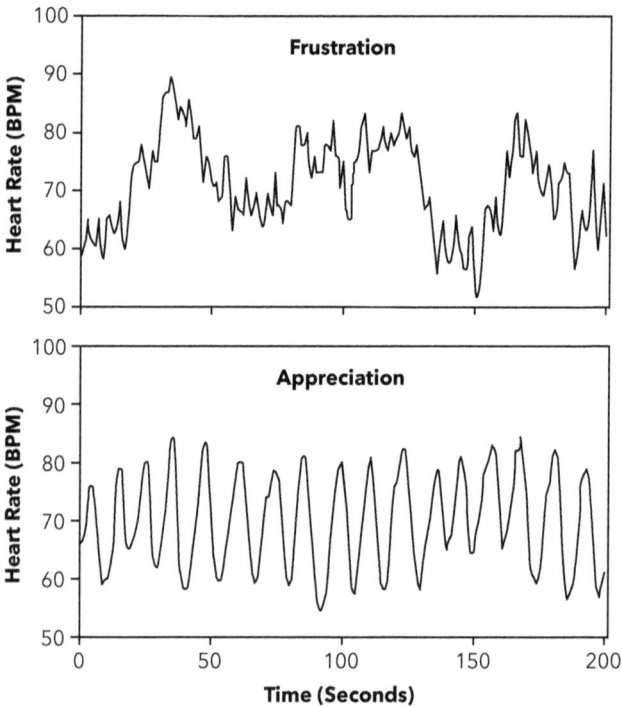

Graph courtesy of HeartMath Institute – www.heartmath.org

When you are in a positive emotion like appreciation, gratitude, and joy, you generate a smooth, sine-like wave that is ordered and harmonious, like beautiful rolling hills and valleys or waves. The two branches of the Autonomic Nervous System (ANS = SNS + PNS) are synchronized and balanced, which directs the body's systems to operate with increased harmony and efficiency. Your adrenals dump DHEA, your feel-good hormone, into your body and you feel clear-headed and vigorous. This is where you want to be when you are in that last minute of the third period of your hockey game, your goalie has been pulled and you need one more goal to tie and go into overtime. You are energized, calm, balanced, focused, and have access to the decision-making centers in your brain because you are in cortical facilitation.

The question of whether our brains have the ability to change through the power of the mind and heart is still being studied by scientists, scholars, and philosophers. If you have the ability to change your own brain's functional and physical anatomy in response to repeated, deliberate, conscious demands, you most certainly have the ability to perform at higher levels.

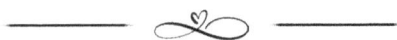

---

*"Since emotional processes can work faster than
the mind, it takes a power stronger than the mind
to bend perception, override emotional circuitry,
and provide us with intuitive feeling instead.
It takes the power of the heart."*

—Doc Childre, HeartMath® Institute founder

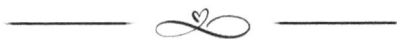

7

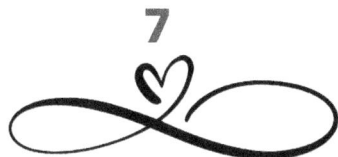

Consciousness Toolbox

TOOL #1:
SEE FAILURE IN A NEW LIGHT

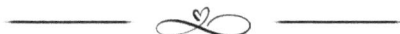

*You may encounter many defeats, but you must
not be defeated. In fact, it may be necessary
to encounter the defeats, so you can know
who you are, what you can rise from,
how you can still come out of it.*

—Maya Angelou

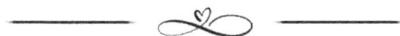

Failure in sport is inevitable. Choosing to see it as negative or bad is optional. If you are going to fulfill your potential as an athlete, you are going to have to redefine failure and learn how to see it in a new light. On many levels, from your brain to the team you play for, failure is a means to an end: of learning and improving. If we encourage ourselves to experiment, take risks, try old things in new ways, and learn from conscious failures, we can deliberately take action towards improving. When you choose to look at failure in this new light, you can take success to a whole new level.

There is no way around "failing," but there is a way to learn how to practice and redefine it. Success and failure are simply perceptions. They are what you have been taught to believe as either desirable or undesirable outcomes. What if every time you failed you viewed it as simply a step towards succeeding? What if you had a coach that encouraged and celebrated failures for a week of practice? Whether you were learning how to walk, swim, throw a ball, or step up to the starting line of a peak event, the path to get you there was full of failures and mistakes. Often, the most successful athletes were willing to be the most vulnerable while learning their sport. They learned how to deal with setbacks and embrace failure rather than be devastated by it.

We are not disturbed by things that happen to us, but by the view that we take of them. How can you possibly move toward success if you choose to get angry or irritated, creating a template of "failure" with thoughts that diminish yourself?

"I never do anything right on the ice."

"I'm such a failure on the field."

"I always do it wrong."

"I suck at pitching."

You may think those kinds of feelings and thoughts may motivate you to do better next time, but negative thoughts only breed or reinforce negative beliefs. Negative responses result in a cascade of negativity that is detrimental to our ability and bodies, and increase the amount of stress in our bodies and lives.

All thoughts that come into our minds are created by us. Those thoughts evoke emotions. They also wire our brains. If you want to get better at your sport, why would you ever choose to see failure as bad or negative and then make it a neural pathway? You would only be working against what you want. Negative thoughts in our minds create a negative physiological response in our brains and bodies. You release stress hormones, your judgment is clouded, your mood diminishes, you feel criticized, and then you expect better performance? Negativity can only trigger a physical, mental, and emotional state that works against you.

—— ∞ ——

*There are no failures, just experiences
and your reaction to them.*

—Tom Krause

—— ∞ ——

Intentionally perceiving failure as an opportunity allows you to access your higher brain, stay in positive emotion, and take action to correct rather than criticize. You can gain as much from your failures as your successes because failures wake you up. Don't allow yourself to be thrown by any circumstances or events you perceive to be failures—your performance and your life are much bigger than any experience you might have. This is Step Five in action: intentionally generating a positive state.

In learning to see failure in a new light or frame of mind, there are a few "four letter words" that we can look at differently: fail, last, loss, beat, fear, weak(ness). All these words have a negative connotation for most of us. What if you changed your view? What if failure was necessary to succeed, that there were lessons in coming last and getting beat? What if loss could be turned into grace? What if fear could be turned into courage? What if your weaknesses could become your strengths?

The one four letter word that is really worse than fail is *quit*. Quitting is one way to ensure that a series of failures do not add up to success. Remember the conscious competence learning model? When you are consciously unskilled, when you know what you don't know, where mistakes must be made to learn, this is where most people give up. You most certainly will not succeed when you quit. I don't know about you, but I would rather fail repeatedly than quit and resign myself to the belief that I "can't" do something. I have been "failing" at handstands for the past couple of years. I work on them every chance I get. There are incremental gains some days and losses on other days. I could quit and say I can't do a handstand, or I can keep attempting, failing, studying, and working toward that new skill. My willingness to endure failure ensures I won't quit. I practice deliberately, keep a beginner's mind and positive emotion, and trust the aggregation of marginal gains.

Learning to change your view is something you can do consciously and repeatedly with practice and dedication. You can learn to not give up at the first sign of discomfort or failure, be less critical and judgmental of yourself, learn how to find solutions more quickly, and have fewer regrets if you do. Failure can take you off course if you don't see that it is pointing you in a new direction.

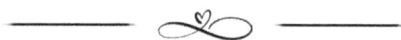

Anyone who has achieved anything great or done anything great to change the world most certainly learned to embrace failure rather than fight it.

—Zoe B.

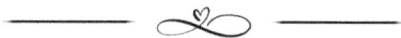

If we didn't fail, how would we learn what is possible or what to do next? The process of learning from our mistakes and failures is of immense value. Taking the attitude of a constant learner is a skill we want to move towards rather than away from. Learning to be comfortable in the discomfort of failing and then moving through and beyond it is a key to success; these are necessary steps on the path to achieving a bigger goal. Consider failing as this: a *First Attempt In Learning*.

Failure shows you what is not working so you can figure out what does work. It is simply feedback and is a necessary part of any success when you're learning to find solutions. "Try, try again" is where that happens. The biggest obstacle to success is an inability to face up to where you are going wrong. Detecting error and adapting to it stops you from going around and around in circles of failure.

Understand that your emotional state affects your ability to learn: if you are in a negative emotional state because you perceive that you are failing, then you will not be able to learn from that failure and move towards success. Remember Step Two towards consciousness: practicing with a beginner's mind. Learning with determination and very little success is most often necessary for great success to happen.

Let's be honest, though. Failure stings. This is why we need to learn how to switch our thinking, stop stamping a weak performance as a *FAILURE!* so quickly and send our mind down a better, more productive path as quickly as possible.

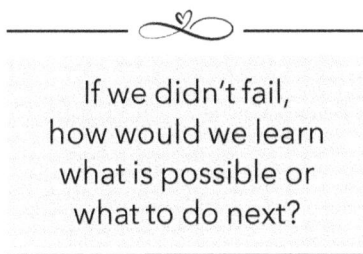

> If we didn't fail, how would we learn what is possible or what to do next?

Shifting your thinking about failure requires new skills. These are four you can start practicing right now that all involve shifting the way you interpret, think, and feel about a situation so you can learn how to enhance your next performance rather than inhibit it.

1. Reframing
2. Cognitive reappraisal
3. Pivoting
4. Plan for the possibility

1. Reframing

Reframing is a technique you can use to change your perspective or the meaning you attach to something. Imagine a beautiful frame around a mediocre picture and notice how that frame makes the picture look great. Or imagine an unattractive frame around a beautiful picture that makes it look mediocre. You can reframe your perspective with awareness, discipline, and practice. Reframing is more than positive thinking and will require you to write a new story, change your perspective, and find meaning in your perceived negative event—giving you a new ability and a sense of hope, clarity, and courage to move forward despite your failures. When you understand that you see a world through a frame, like the film in the projector, you become free to try something new.

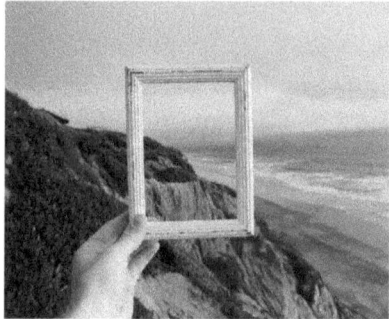

In 1968, American high jumper Dick Fosbury changed the way high jumpers around the world achieve the great heights they do today. Back then, his technique seemed unusual. He used his "Fosbury Flop" to flop over the bar backwards and win an Olympic gold medal. Prior to that, the belief was that you went over the bar forwards with the Western Roll. Before the Western Roll came into practice, when there were no big mats to fall onto, high jumpers scissored their legs over the bar and landed on their feet. Seeing a completely different technique meet with such success required that the technique and the belief around it shifted. By the 1972 Olympics, most elite high jumpers in the world had reframed their belief system and perspective on how to achieve greater heights.

On May 6th, 1954, Roger Banister became the first person to run a mile in less than four minutes. Up until that point in history, the prevailing belief was that it was impossible. There was no way the human body could withstand what it would require to run that fast. Up until that day, Roger Banister had not achieved his goal of breaking that barrier. He had "failed" in his attempts and could have given up with the excuse that it was impossible. He chose to defy the psychological barrier and general belief that had been imposed. Using scientific methods and studying the mechanics of running, he proved his theory correct. The frame around the mile time shifted. In that same year, 30 other runners followed Banister's lead.

Banister and Fosbury reframed what was possible. Through their determination to challenge conventional wisdom, to try new things, to experiment, to be the first to do something, to figure out a way, and to be alert and awake enough and not fuss about failing. This applies today.

When you reframe, you actually work towards changing your beliefs. You can use this in Step Three towards consciousness, where you take your inventory. Reframing is straightforward and helps you see the insanity in the framework of beliefs and thoughts you built long ago. Going through the process step-by-step and seeing the finished frame can help you identify and manage your emotions and thoughts. This process is based on Karim Benammar's book *Reframing: The Art of Thinking Differently,* which outlines four steps to a more conscious way of looking at how you think, what beliefs support that thinking, and the transformation that's possible when you are able to change what passes through your mind. (Benammar, 2012).

THE FOUR STEP PROCESS TO REFRAMING

a. Determine what your current position is. This is your core belief.

b. Analyze this core belief. What are the reasons you think that? Come up with "supporting beliefs" and pick the four most important ones.

c. Force yourself to construct the opposite of these supporting beliefs by finding antonyms and grammatical opposites. This is the artificial element in the technique, the way to jolt your thinking. Come up with variations on these opposites until you find extreme formulations. If these extremes are ludicrous and laughable, you can be certain you have pushed yourself outside of your frame.

d. Consider your opposite supporting beliefs and suspend disbelief by asking what would happen if they were all true. What reframed core belief would this lead to?

Reframing is one of the favorite tools in the toolbox; it feels physically liberating for people to force themselves to think differently. This is especially true for people who are experienced in sports, because they have completely internalized underlying assumptions. It is eye-opening and freeing to be asked to take a very different perspective. It makes people feel "unstuck" where they were previously part of conventional wisdom thinking.

2. Cognitive Reappraisal

Cognitive reappraisal is a technique to calm and harness your emotions. It starts with recognizing that you have patterns of thought that you have fallen into that can be changed, just like you can change patterns of movement in your sport. Intentionally generating a positive state of coherence (Step Five) is consistent with this technique.

You believe things because you think they are true, but the truth is, you believe things because you've practiced the thought.

Becoming conscious of those patterns (Step One) is necessary in order to change them. You must first recognize and own your negative response, and then practice reinterpreting the situation to either reduce the severity of that negative response or exchange it for a more positive one. Challenging negative patterns and the associated thoughts and emotions allows them to be restructured to allow adaptive thinking and problem solving.

Here's the thing: performance does not improve by chance. Performance improves by change, and we cannot change what we don't notice. Your performance does not change who you are; who you are changes your performance.

Using the cognitive reappraisal technique, you will be able to notice triggers that fire up emotions and inhibit performance and then learn how to manage their intensity to productively deal with whatever triggered you to begin with. Emotions start with your perception of a stimulus within a context. You may be on the starting line of a big race that you feel pressure to win. Then, you appraise that stimulus' emotional significance, and this triggers an affective, physiological, and behavioral response. You feel anxiety and fear of failing to reach that expectation. Cognitive reappraisals target that appraisal stage and involve changing one's interpretations or appraisals of affective stimuli. Instead of feeling fear and anxiety, you feel confident and calm in knowing that no matter how you perform, you will learn something from it.

We all assign meaning to situations based on our past experience and our beliefs. The way we think about situations will elicit an emotional response. Different thinking will produce different emotions, and different emotions will produce different thoughts. Our subjective appraisal of an event, what it means and what its significance is, rather than the event itself, is what leads to our emotional reaction.

Consider this emotion-thought feedback loop:

You and your teammates are playing the best you have all year in the championship hockey game. Your team is down by one goal. There is one minute left in the game. You get the puck and a breakaway to score the goal to tie the game and bring you into overtime. You shoot and miss the net. Your immediate thought is, "Because of me, we lost the championship." You have personalized the loss by thinking that you deserve the majority of the blame, while discounting your teammates' responsibility. You feel awful, frustrated, perhaps even angry with yourself. You have discounted the positive 59 minutes of the game and focused on the one negative.

Take a moment to consider another perspective. Reappraise the missed goal. Become conscious of the way different thoughts will evoke different feelings.

"I always choke under pressure."

"The team is going to be so disappointed in me."

Or:

"I practiced hard and did my best."

Every thought and feeling you may have about a single event may be valid to some extent, and you can have multiple and even conflicting feelings at the same time—that makes us human. When you are more fully conscious, however, you can see there is not just one way for any of us to evaluate a situation and try to make sense of it. As competitors, we can see that we are often harder on ourselves than others are on us. It's almost as if we want to punish and berate ourselves before others have a chance to do so. *This helps nothing.* Instead, we can learn to create a feedback loop that brings us to a place where we can learn rather than wallow.

Reappraisals are not a gloss of positive thinking smeared over a failure, but are conscious, valid, reality-based ways of looking at and redefining the situation. They allow other ways that make sense of a situation to co-exist with the more emotional appraisal.

"That was a great game. I did my best and accept this outcome."

"My teammates are awesome, and I am grateful for the season we had together. Making it to the championship game was amazing."

You may be rolling your eyes, but *losing badly is not winning.* If you didn't win the championship game, you can still learn to manage your emotions so that you haven't deepened the negative feedback loop the next time the pressure is on. When I watch any team deal with a loss, it tells me more about their performance than anything. The more negative or blaming the players are, the more potential there is for them to work with their cognitive strategies. You don't ignore what went wrong, but you don't look at it hyper-critically and negatively and think you don't have the power to change. Athletes who lose badly think they "should" have won. Their ego gets in the way of figuring out how to do better next time. Athletes who lose well understand how to do better next time. Their humility and perspective allow them to learn from their losses.

It will be difficult at first, but you can at least begin to be conscious of other possibilities and trigger positive emotions rather than negative. Personally, it is easier for me to evoke positive emotions in negative situations, rather than positive thought. Joy or gratitude for what was good always helps me deal with what I perceive to be bad and, as a result, perform better the next time.

Cognitive reappraisal is really a technique to regulate and gain mastery of your emotions. The ability to manage your emotional state is what separates the elites from the rest. Successful athletes will always redirect the old, familiar course of negative thoughts, feelings, and situations to their advantage. They know how to adjust the interpretive lens of their mind. If you learn how to change your emotional response from negative to positive by reinterpreting your meaning of the stimulus, you will be learning to make opportunities out of obstacles, to see potential in losses, and to experience breakdowns as breakthroughs.

3. Pivoting

Pivoting is another technique you can use to adjust that interpretive lens of your mind. Doubts and thoughts of failures from your past can come into your mind and can have a powerful and negative affect on your performance in the present. You can consciously, deliberately, and

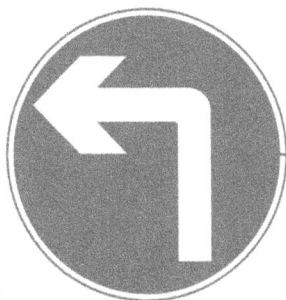

swiftly pivot those doubts and thoughts in the complete opposite direction, and in doing so, choose to change the effect they have on you and your performance. Learning this technique gives you power in the moment to choose a positive outcome rather than allowing a previous negative one to affect your performance.

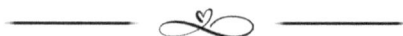

The pessimist sees difficulty in every opportunity.
The optimist sees opportunity in every difficulty.

—Winston Churchill

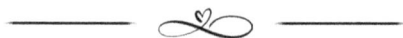

Consider that you are playing soccer against a team you have never beaten before. During the warm up, you watch the other team and start to think about how much better they are than you and how you are going to lose yet again. You just hope that they don't win by more than 10 goals this time.

So, how do you pivot in that situation?

The first thing you can do is pivot your attention. I like to call it "keeping your head in your own boat." If you are more concerned about what is going on with your competitors than with yourself and your own team, you are giving away your power and energy. Keep your focus on the warm-up of your team. Think about how hard you have been practicing this past week and how your teammates are skilled and working well together.

In this way, you can be in the present moment rather than the end of the game by allowing yourself to detach from outcome. The game hasn't been played yet and you have already predicted a slaughter. Predicting failure and loss can be your strong suit if you continually believe what you think. Pivoting those thoughts to playing well and scoring goals despite the score is the next step in diminishing the power of past losses in your current game. Deliberately choosing a thought based on your desire to win (where you want to go) rather than your fear of losing (where you don't want to go) allows you to take control of the moment and of your mental game. It takes practice to consciously choose a thought that is consistent with what you desire, rather than allowing one that hijacks it.

This powerful change in the direction of your thinking will fundamentally alter the direction of your sport—and, not incidentally, your whole life. Shifting your thoughts to what you desire hinges on your cognitive awareness. Recognize a negative thought as soon as it enters your mind, reappraise to rebuild a positive outcome, then redirect your thoughts and emotions towards success.

4. Plan for the Possibility of Failure

You can be intentionally ready for success, but intention and feeling ready doesn't necessarily mean that you will be successful. Anything can happen as you reach for your goals. Being ready to deal with the unexpected by having a plan can help you build confidence to defend against the fear of failure. If you confront the possibility and fear of failure head-on, you forge strong skills and develop competence to deal with it, along with a hard-won kind of competence and resilience.

There is a big difference between thinking you are going to fail and preparing for it in case you do. Thinking you will fail is discouraging, while preparing for it encourages progress. Recognizing the possibility may help you reduce complacency and keep you on track to your desired outcome.

There is a term in psychology called "implementation intention." (Gollwitzer, 1999). When you have a goal in place, it provides a strategy to develop new habits and behaviors to deal with failure before it happens. Psychologists use the "if-then" plan you make beforehand about how you intend to act. If or when I meet up with an obstacle to achieving my goal, I will take this action (whatever your plan is) to overcome it. It is knowing ahead of time what to do if you start to veer off course and knowing precisely what veering off course actually looks like for you. If you don't determine ahead of time what it would take for you to quit or what failure looks like, you may quit prematurely.

You can look ahead to your goal and also practice how to get back on course if you veer off. What would it take for you to quit? When you set parameters and predetermine where your edge is, you reduce your chances of quitting prematurely. Most people will quit before they reach their actual ability if they haven't decided how to get beyond obstacles that are simply opportunities to test limits.

In her book *Rethinking Positive Thinking*, Gabrielle Oettingen talks about implementation intentions and mental contrasting, and describes a four-step process she calls WOOP: Wish, Outcome, Obstacle, Plan. Having a desired outcome and identifying possible obstacles to achieving it is very different from just thinking positively. (Oettingen, 2014). After you imagine that positive outcome, mental contrasting is identifying things standing in the way of your goals that could lead to failure. You are then connecting your goals with your current reality. When you do that, you can practice behaviors to overcome those obstacles and achieve the success you desire. It's about visualizing your goal and also imagining the speed bumps, potholes, dead ends, and detours built in along the way, and learning to deal with them before you hit them. Mentally contrasting a desired future with impending reality can activate expectation of success: when expectations are high, people fully commit and pursue their goals; when expectations of success are low, people postpone or abandon the fulfillment of their wishes. (Oettingen, 2014).

One of my favorite athletes is Diana Nyad who, at 64, became the first person to swim from Cuba to the US without a shark cage. She had failed four times before succeeding in 2013. She never gave up her dream, continually planning over and over again how to deal with everything from doubters and fatigue to venomous jellyfish and currents. She shared her understanding of overcoming what failure looks like in the book *Find A Way*, especially her biggest life lesson:

just because someone says something is impossible, doesn't mean it is true. "You can do all the computations you want as to why this is impossible and this can't be done," she told ABC News. "But don't ever tell me what the parameters of the human spirit are. We have no idea how powerful our hearts and our souls are. We only know how limited our muscles are." (ABC News, 2015).

Seeing failure in a new light by practicing these simple techniques will help you:

- Stay in the moment, out of the past and future
- Focus on your strengths, not your weaknesses
- Control what you can, accept what you cannot
- Do your best, not your "perfect"

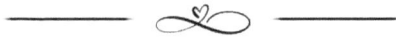

There is much to be said for failure. It is so much more interesting than success.

—Max Beerbohm

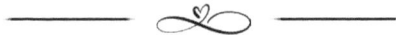

TOOL #2:
GET TO KNOW YOUR AMYGDALA

As you move into consciousness and work towards making changes in your sport and your life, you may experience your own resistance to those changes even though you "know" they will help you perform better. As talked about earlier in the book, the "consciously unskilled" stage, when you know what you don't know, is the stage where most people give up. Factor in your amygdala to that change and it will require even more awareness and desire to make the changes you know will help you perform better. Your amygdala, in your mid-brain, is where that resistance resides and it is driven by the wired-in and programmed reactions we have to fear. It is really your *unconscious* fear center. Becoming conscious is where performance lies in your brain anatomy. You must make a commitment to consciously respond instead of automatically reacting to the situation. That is the only way to create positive and lasting changes in your experience.

Many of you athletes may ride your bike and know what the saddle feels like under your pelvis. Sometimes it is comfortable for the short term, but over the long haul, you get saddle sores, blisters, or even back pain. Just as the wiring of our brain may be comfortable for the short term, over the long term, it may do more harm than good. I had a seat mapping done for my road bike after many miles of discomfort I needed to address. We discovered I was sitting heavy in my right hip, my handlebars were too low, my saddle was at the wrong angle, and as a result, I was not accessing the power available to me. After making corrections to my bike position, it was immediately apparent to me how I had been adapting to a poor position with no awareness as to what was possible with the bike fitted to my body. Just as you can get more power from your body with the right alignment and position, you can get more power from your mind when you come into consciousness and map or sculpt your brain to tap into your potential.

Sculpting Your Performance

We can actually use the mind to change the brain.
The simple truth is that how we focus our attention,
how we intentionally direct the flow of energy
and information through our neural circuits, can
directly alter the brain's activity and its structure.
The key is to know the steps toward using our
awareness in ways that promote well-being.

—Rick Hanson, Ph.D.

That shaping of your brain is what scientists have called neuro-plasticity since the late 1960s. Every thought you think or don't think, every bit of stimulus that you perceive, and all the information you take in or learn makes or changes connections between neurons. Your life will shape your brain until you learn how to use your brain to shape your life. As the saying goes, "You are what you think."

We've been talking about developing important new tools, and learning how to work with your stimulus/reaction patterns is one of them. In order to learn how to use this tool, you need to meet and train your brain—or at least one part of it, the amygdala. The way you respond to stimulus today has been hardwired by your past. If you find yourself throwing up the night before every big game or race, you have learned to *re*act to some fear you have of performance. Your amygdala recognizes that stimulus and reacts to it with a physiological response that literally makes you sick. That pattern of stimulus-response is habitual and unconscious, and you may believe it to be inevitable and unchangeable.

Not so.

Learning to work with that pattern to shift it is something you can do to enhance your performance instead of spending a night vomiting and inhibiting it. Change will allow you to find out what you are capable of on race or game day without that conditioned response ruining the night before the event.

You can learn to respond/act rather than react to situations, and learning to do just that can have a huge impact on your ability to perform. Reaction is an instinct driven by your reptilian brain that sometimes can save your life. It can also be a habitual skill, pattern, or behavior that is so automatic you don't even have to think about it. Response/action is a conscious choice using our more evolved cortex and intelligence, along with developing our ability to observe ourselves and develop an *inner coach.*

Learning to respond/act rather than react may sound easy, but it will challenge not just your mind/thinking—it will also challenge your brain. A neurological rewiring or re-routing will be necessary. Learning how to change your reactive patterns to stimuli that affect your performance in a negative way is another way to become a more conscious athlete. Understanding how to bypass your amygdala so it doesn't hijack your ability is key to making that change. Knowing how your amygdala works is where you begin.

Your amygdala is a small, almond-shaped structure deep in your brain's temporal lobes. It is where your "fight, flight, or freeze" response lives. It is always on watch in our brains. It observes all situations and determines whether they are harmless or threatening. This warning system is essential to your survival, sensitive, and always ready to alert you to what it perceives as a threat. It is our autonomic response to fear. We can condition ourselves with regards to fear. There is an associative learning process where we learn by repeated experiences to fear something, and as a result, our neural circuitry actually changes to produce a fear response.

If you were bitten by a dog when you were a child, chances are you learned to fear all dogs. Other children don't fear the same trigger because their amygdalae have not had the same experience as yours. Your memory of that event will go beyond just the bite. You will remember other factors associated with other sense organs. The kind of dog, the sound of it barking, who you were with, a song that may have been playing in the background, the smell of the park you were in: all those things were stored into your memory bank to be forever associated with that dog biting you. Problems arise when the response to the memory becomes oversensitive. Just going back to that park may trigger an intense response even if there are no dogs around.

When your amygdala perceives a stimulus, it sends the information to other areas of the brain. If it considers the stimulus a threat, it tells the hypothalamus to release stress hormones that trigger a fight or flight response. (Harvard Health Publishing, 2020). When those hormones are released, emotional memories and feelings associated with the stimulus are imprinted and put into the long-term memory banks of the fascia of our bodies. Oxygen is moved to your arms and legs and away from your brain. It sets up a file of sorts that can be indexed with many experiences associated with the events. When your emotional system learns something, it requires awareness to unlearn. The limbic system of our brains holds our memories and will respond to the memory of the past situation, not the reality of the current situation.

When there is a trigger of a strong emotion followed by an automatic or knee-jerk reaction during an intense moment in sport, there can be feelings of regret when the reaction inhibits performance. Reacting to the past rather than the current situation can impact your present ability, no matter how fast, skilled, talented, strong, and ready you are. Imagine the best player on your women's high school volleyball team is ready to serve the game-winning point when her ex-boyfriend walks into the gym. They recently had a very emotional breakup. Her face immediately flushes, and she is angry he has shown up. Seeing her ex-boyfriend has triggered her amygdala to react to the emotions associated with him. The ball goes into the net, and she gets mad at herself for allowing him to affect her so much. Her amygdala has hijacked her ability to perform. Understanding how that process happens and how to ensure it doesn't happen again can be invaluable knowledge for athletes and coaches in the heat of the moment.

At this point, your amygdala is not a part of your brain that is under your conscious control. It's a spring-loaded trap that snaps-to when an unexpected person or event triggers it.

The fact is, your brain and your body both get hijacked when a sensory signal comes into the body through any or all of your senses: sight, smell, touch, sound, or taste. The thalamus, which filters all input to your brain, decides if and where the stimulus goes. If it decides to process the stimulus, the signal goes through your amygdala, which quickly searches its memory banks to decide whether the signal is an emergency when it compares it to past experiences. Once declared to be an emergency, the hypothalamus and limbic/reptilian brain both go into survival mode. All the while, the thalamus has also sent the signal to the cortex to be processed, but it is a much slower pathway than the one to the amygdala. Emotions are already in charge, hormones have been released, and rational thinking is overridden. A fight or flight response has been triggered by a park with no dog to bite you or an ex-boyfriend who hasn't said a word to you.

Considering that we are human beings who want to live and avoid harm, it is necessary for us to have a strong response to stimulus. If there is a car moving towards you as you cross the street, you start to run to get out of its way. That is a good thing. The brain is wired to sense danger and react to that danger to keep us alive. It will constantly scan our inner and outer environments for threats. We have survived as a species because our brains are really wired more for avoiding than approaching. Negative experiences are more likely to threaten your survival than positive ones. If you fail to notice a car speeding through an intersection while you are running, you are less likely to experience the joy of taking a hot shower afterwards. To put it in stark and real terms, there will be more sporting events for you to enjoy only if you live to participate in them. Thankfully, we've been unconsciously conditioned with this response all because a small part of our brain has been trained for millions of years to keep us "in the game," as it were—that is, the game of life.

Knowing that this part of our brain has been conditioned for survival, we can see that it can also be conditioned for other behaviors.

Let's see how we can exert conscious influence over it. The tools that can help to exert that influence include:

1. Practice acting instead of reacting.
2. Know your triggers and emotional intelligence.
3. Tiptoe around your amygdala.
4. Practice caution and curiosity instead of fight or flight.
5. Force-feed success.

1. Act. Don't React.

One simple way to practice consciousness is to understand stimulus and response so that we can understand what happens to us and how we respond to what happens, or respond to what we *perceive* has happened. We can have knee-jerk or unconscious reactions, or we can act with mindfulness, consciousness. In his book *First Things First,* Stephen Covey reminds us that there is a space between stimulus and response. (Covey, 1996). We have the power in that space to consciously choose how we deal with what happens to us in our lives other than to simply react in a way that is old and familiar and maybe even harmful to ourselves and others. We can choose to rewire and reshape our brain rather than have it unconsciously shape our lives and our performance. What affects us is the *meaning* we attach to an event.

Learning to change interpretations and meaning can make you bulletproof.

Your perception is how your brain processes sensory information. As the brain has learned to anticipate and predict what it thinks is going to happen next, it has built perceptual filters that select and organize awareness based on previous experience. Those filters shape what you focus on and influence what information goes into your brain. Some filters are good. Those filters can help make things more predictable for us in our sport. For example, scanning the field of opponents in a soccer game filters our options to select what we need to react to. Filters continually reinforce themselves, which means we think what we perceive through them is accurate and complete. When we only see what conforms to our existing beliefs, we are really conforming our perceptions to fit with our beliefs. If those filters become too rigid, you will not have access to that beginner's mind and will limit your ability to grow as an athlete. Rigid filters set expectations, create biases, and limit beliefs that all close you off to possibility.

Perception is an aspect of consciousness that you will want to expand. If you use the broader lens of "it seems" or "it appears" to describe what you are perceiving, it leaves a space to explore other possibilities of those interpretations and meanings you would previously not have considered. From that platform of discovery and creativity, you bring the openness to the anything-is-possible mindset. When you change your language from, "We never win a game" to "It seems as if we never win a game," you are deliberately and consciously reframing your perception of never winning instead of unconsciously believing what you have always told yourself. This is where you can step into that beginner's mind with a "let's try" attitude to practice something you may not have considered before.

Possibly the best-known law of Newton's Three Laws of Motion tells us that for every action, there is an equal and opposite reaction. As human beings, we can behave according to that law or we can step into that space, that consciousness, and make a choice to not react, but to act.

Everything can be taken from a man
but the last of human freedoms— the ability
to choose one's attitude in a given set
of circumstances, to choose one's way.

—Viktor Frankl

One of the qualities of humanness is our ability to observe ourselves. We can look at what we believe, how we behave, believe, move, adapt, respond, and feel. We can be separate and observe ourselves even though we are ourselves. The potential for growth is in that space, that awareness, that consciousness. As an athlete, you can step into that space as your own *inner coach* and develop a deep understanding of how you operate and create new ways to be the best you possible.

**Linking reaction to its source action
requires a conscious application of awareness.**

Stimulus (what happens to you)	**Space** between stimulus and response	Response (what you do)
Event	Power (consciousness) Activate awareness/ inner coach	Act (conscious) React (unconscious)
Being passed by someone in your age group	"This is not about how fast they are or how slow I am. It seems like I am being passed."	Conscious act: smile Unconscious reaction: get angry and speed up

The cycle of action and reaction is very deeply ingrained in our behavioral patterns. Most of the time, we don't even recognize it for what it is. We ride the merry-go-round of reactivity, oblivious that we are even on it. The first step is to identify the reaction, especially to something we perceive to be negative—which, in turn, arouses negative emotions. If we get passed in the last mile of the run by someone in our age group, we may get angry. We must be able to look into the space between being passed and getting angry and clearly recognize that anger has nothing to do with the person who passed you. It has everything to do with your expectations of yourself and your perception of the situation. Taking a step away from yourself and letting the conscious athlete inside you make the decisions will help you perform to your potential rather than be driven by fear that may never allow you to reach that potential.

When we act out of fear, we are not really acting, but *re*acting. It takes no rational thought, just a knee-jerk response that is often one you would not have in calmer, more sane moments. Fear-based reactions to non-life-threatening situations are never good decisions. You may go through a process that you call "thinking," but if it is fear and reaction-based, it is not a clear, conscious choice and will lead you down a path you most likely will regret.

There is a network of neural pathways that connect your amygdala to your "thinking brain," or your neocortex. It allows you to reflect on your feelings and think before you react. When you are in a perceived crisis, however, those pathways get bypassed and impulse overrides reason. Neuro-logic goes out the window and neuro-emotion wins. When you succumb to road rage or yell at your spouse over an innocent remark, your amygdala is hijacking your brain and your knee-jerk response to a perception rather than the reality creates havoc in your body. Although it may not be easy to maintain such awareness and coach yourself, just like when you first started down the road of your sport, you will have to practice. Learning to find that gap in the fabric of time between what happens to you and whether you choose to stop and consider what to do next can become a valuable opportunity to choose to act rather than react. In choosing and practicing a more aware response based on the values we want to enact in our lives, we may move closer to the person we strive to be. If you consider yourself to be a compassionate, caring human being, how can you be angry at the person who just passed you in the race? That split-second of awareness doesn't change that you were passed, but it does remind you that you are the incredible human being you believe yourself to be.

---

*I am convinced that life is 10% what
happens to me and 90% how I react to it.*

—Scipio Africanus

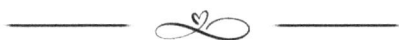

---

2. Know Your Triggers: Raise Your EQ and Your Results

---

*Emotional intelligence is a way of recognizing,
understanding, and choosing how we think, feel,
and act. It shapes our interactions with others and
our understanding of ourselves. It defines how
and what we learn; it allows us to set priorities;
it determines the majority of our daily actions.
Research suggests it is responsible for as much
as 80 percent of the "success" in our lives.*

—Joshua Freedman

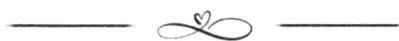

In 1983, Howard Gardner looked at how intelligence tests were
lacking with reference to measuring true intelligence. He proposed
a theory that true intelligence requires you to consider eight different intelligences accounting for a broader range of human potential.
(Gardner, 2011). The term "emotional intelligence," EI or EQ, was
coined and defined as the capacity to recognize your own and others'
emotions, to discriminate between and label different emotions, and
to use that information to guide thinking and behavior. A big part of

emotional intelligence is being able to feel an emotion without having to act on it. As mentioned before, what separates elite athletes from the rest of us is their ability to manage their emotional state under stress. They have a high awareness of their strengths, limitations, and how their emotions and behaviors create their sport results. Having a high EQ can be learned and practiced no matter what age or ability you are. People who lack emotional intelligence don't deal well with change; learning to make changes before it's too painful not to is something we could all benefit from.

You may have a high IQ and understand cognitively what needs to be done to enhance your performance, and also have a low EQ that hijacks or overrides that intelligence. Even when you know what you "could" do, it doesn't mean you will—especially when you are overwhelmed by what you perceive to be stress. Increasing your awareness of and harnessing negative emotions that hijack your ability gives you the opportunity to choose productive, positive emotions that allow access to your ability.

Emotions control your actions, your behavior, and your thoughts. Emotions affect your physical body as much as your body affects how you feel and think. Athletes who don't address their emotions set themselves up not only for a poor performance, but perhaps for a serious illness. Negative, fear-based emotions like anxiety, frustration, anger, and depression that are felt but not released can cause chemical reactions in your brain and body that are very different from the chemicals released when you feel positive emotions such as happiness, confidence, gratitude, and joy.

There is an undeniable connection between your emotions and your physiology. Every emotion sparks or triggers a distinctive physiological reaction. For the first time, researchers in Finland recently mapped emotions that detail where we feel them in our bodies. (PNAS, 2013). It showed that all humans show a similar genetically coded physiological response to emotions. Mapping where psychology affects our physiology gives clear routes to those responses happening in our body. Having awareness of the emotional impact on the corresponding area of our body is a powerful opportunity to navigate without getting lost. That map is a direct route to accessing more power from our body and mind with the deliberate awareness and choice of emotion. Perception of those emotions and the physiological response they trigger can play an important role in learning how to generate consciously-felt emotions.

Your body has been programmed to deal with different situations that arise in your emotional life. Happiness increases the body's energy levels, while sadness does the opposite, slowing down your metabolism and manifesting most clearly in tears. Your heart may feel sadness as an ache, or race when it feels fear. Anger floods your brain with catecholamine hormones that stimulate your nervous system and put you in a general state of alert; your blood pressure goes up and your muscles contract. When your fight or flight response is chronically set off by your perceived stress and anxiety, it can lead to headaches, cramps, or insomnia along with more serious physical issues such as heart disease, colitis, and gastrointestinal disorders. Imagine what learning to manage your emotions under stress can do to your performance, along with enhancing your overall health.

If you recall, the Fifth Step in consciousness is intentional or deliberate generation of a positive state of physiological coherence—positive emotion. You can learn to follow the map of positive emotion and avoid ending up in a place you really don't want to be without understanding how you got there. When you allow those fear-based negative emotions to run wild in your body and brain, you have put your amygdala in the driver's seat. If your life is in danger, that is a good driver to have, but if your fear is self-imposed, that driver will take you down a road as its passenger. You may want to go in a different direction than your amygdala is taking you, but you have no power to do that once it is at the wheel. If you want better results on race day, don't allow your amygdala even on the road/court/field or in the game.

Being aware of your emotions is the first step towards being able to manage them. In the space between stimulus and response, you have the opportunity to practice being your own coach and be conscious and aware of whether you are reacting or acting. Think about a time when you were performing and you were particularly stressed. Perhaps it was a big game with a championship on the line, or it was the first time you stepped up to an international stage. Maybe it was your first time away from home competing with no support from friends and family, or you had experienced some personal trauma prior to your race. Was it easy for you to think clearly and make decisions? Most likely not.

Being outside our comfort zones can put our brain on alert. Your brain usually manages feelings and thinking at the same time quite well, but when you feel stressed, your ability to do both becomes compromised and hijacked by your amygdala getting involved. The only person who can change what you feel is you. Thinking that something outside of you will change your feelings is only a temporary fix. Winning on a big stage may feel good when it happens. If you feel unworthy of that win because of a belief system operating under the radar of your awareness, that fix will wear off. Eventually, you will still feel unworthy, despite your success.

To improve your EQ, you must first be aware of your emotions. Practice with your inner coach, noticing and labeling how you feel. As discussed in the "taking inventory" step, your reactions may be found buried deep in quadrant two of the Johari Window, your blind spot, and it will most certainly take some digging to bring them into consciousness.

Once you know how you feel, look towards understanding why you feel that way. The key to emotional intelligence comes when you learn to manage those emotions and develop strategies to change them. Self-awareness and self-regulation are key. Responding in a way that enhances performance rather than inhibits it is dependent on becoming more emotionally intelligent and taking responsibility for those emotions. Your attitude towards your emotions, yourself, and your team can improve by realizing that you can tiptoe around and undo the hijack perpetrated by your amygdala.

Stimulus ➔ Emotion ➔ **Filter** ➔ Interpret ➔ Behavior

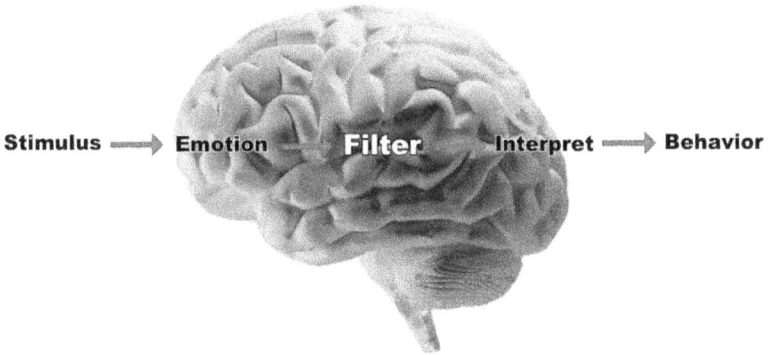

Research has shown that psychological skills facilitate athletic performance. Relaxation training, positive thought control, self-regulation, imagery, concentration, energy control, self-monitoring, and goal setting are all traits that have been correlated with athletic performance. Many of those traits reflect emotional intelligence.

It is very important to understand that emotional intelligence is not the opposite of intelligence, it is not the triumph of heart over head—it is the unique intersection of both.

—David Caruso

---

3. Tiptoe Around Your Amygdala

Practicing small, easily-achievable tiptoe steps (the Kaizen method) will allow your cortex to start working and creating new pathways for the desired changes you want to make. New memories can be made, stored, and associated with positive emotions that will circumvent the brain's built-in resistance to change or being outside of its comfort zone. You may not be able to change your emotions immediately, but you can learn how to spend less time in them and in your hijacked state. The Kaizen method is based on small, incremental, continual improvement consistent with the aggregation of marginal gains practice. You improve by taking incremental steps, as small as one percent a day. Small improvements will compound on the achievement of each day. You will not see improvement at first, but over time, there will be positive and profound change.

You may trigger the amygdala with a sense of threat if you set your goals too big when you are trying to change a pattern of movement, behavior, or thought, or when you're perhaps trying to build a new pattern of communication or play with your teammates. Emotional reactions will inhibit the desired change and have a debilitating effect. The fight component may present itself by rejecting the change; avoidance of the new ideas may be revealed with passive or active opposition.

When you introduce something new to your brain or your team, consider setting the vision of the change and then outline small, manageable Kaizen steps to get there. That way, you tiptoe around the amygdala and don't trigger unnecessary distress. Kaizen trumps the amygdala and goals are attained in a non-threatening, unresisted way.

Consider this step-by-step process when faced with a change you want to make:

1. Notice any negative or limiting emotion and breath.
2. Label the emotion and slowly breathe it out.
3. Replace that emotion with a positive one (my personal favorite is gratitude) and breathe it in. Take power away from your amygdala and come into your higher consciousness.
4. Continue until you feel your fight or flight response diminish.
5. Smile and congratulate yourself.

6. When you are out of the stressful situation, take some time to consider where in your past you may have learned to respond negatively and why.
7. Explore the possibility of creating new wiring with these new techniques.
8. Consciously practice the new pathways/emotions/thoughts the next time you find yourself in that situation.

You *can* rewire your brain and your physical responses with different techniques that make the most sense to you. Find ways around the fight-or-flight response you are wired to use. Regulate yourself. Use imagery by creating a mental movie in your mind of success. Increase your concentration and focus. Control your energy expenditure and level. Learning to relax under pressure and choosing not just positive, but also productive thoughts and emotions is how you will enhance athletic performance and improve your emotional intelligence.

When I was a new paddler learning how to stay upright in the tippy kayaks I wanted to race in, I panicked when I saw motorboats. They would speed by me, creating wash and waves that often tipped me over and sent me swimming to the shore. More experienced paddlers around me knew what to do. They told me, "Cindy, you love to paddle through wash." I told them I did not. They told me to say it whenever a situation came up when a motorboat threw wash at me. Lo and behold, I learned to love wash, stay in the boat, and re-pattern my old thoughts and emotions to enhance my sport rather than give up on it. Taking my amygdala out of the equation with positive thoughts, a positive emotion, and relaxing upon sighting a motorboat was the way for me to tiptoe around my fight or "tip" response that previously had hijacked my ability to paddle. To this day, I find myself smiling and saying "I love to paddle through wash" when I meet up with any situation that challenges me.

4. Practice Caution and Curiosity

Curiosity is not a sin... But we should exercise caution with our curiosity... Yes, indeed.

—J.K. Rowling

Curiosity is involved in the process of learning in all aspects of human development. Inquisitive thinking, exploration, and investigation will help you when you want to acquire knowledge and skill. When you consider that anything is possible, exploring possibilities is a way to move to new levels. Curiosity sparks the driving force behind developments in sport and science. Curiosity draws you forward.

Caution is curiosity's teammate. It means paying careful attention to the probable effects of an act, so that failure or harm may be avoided. It is being prudent and wary in regards to danger. Caution yanks you back into the moment. Caution allows you to plot your actions in your mind's eye, to anticipate how your reactions may affect your performance, and to rehearse for adversity.

Practicing caution in tandem with curiosity is another way to get around your amygdala. Although we are wired for fight, flight, or freeze when we perceive fear, we can instead learn to choose caution and curiosity and stay in our logical, rational, highly-skilled brains. You may not be winning your tennis match, but instead of allowing doubt and fear to hijack the possibility of that win, you can use your mind and your emotions to rationally start developing a new game plan that moves you in the direction of confidence and hope.

Instead of fight, flight, or freeze when you are not in imminent danger, caution and curiosity are one tool for you to learn as an athlete to enhance your performance. In his book *An Astronaut's Guide to Life on Earth*, Chris Hadfield speaks to the skills he learned as an astronaut to make the impossible possible. "It takes years of serious, sustained effort because you need to build a new knowledge base, develop your physical capabilities, and dramatically expand your technical skill set. But the most important thing you need to change? Your mind." (Hadfield, 2013). What Hadfield learned as an astronaut to build those skills is what athletes can learn and use also.

Hadfield's astronaut training taught him to develop a new set of skills that overrode his instincts. Instead of responding to a fire alarm on a spaceship with the survival mode adrenaline rush, he bypassed the amygdala and its associated emotions, looked to understand what was going wrong, and figured out how to fix it. A fire had to be approached with caution and curiosity in order to survive. "Rehearsing for catastrophe has made me positive that I have the problem solving skills to deal with tough situations and come out the other side smiling… This has greatly reduced the mental and emotional clutter that worrying produces, those random thoughts that hijack your brain at three o'clock in the morning." (Hadfield, 2013).

I realized that the words you hear shape you,
but the most important words you'll ever hear in
your entire life are the words you say to yourself.

—Marissa Peer

I was not rehearsing for any catastrophe in 2000 when I raced at Ironman New Zealand. I was rehearsing for a long day that potentially had some tough conditions for me to deal with. My mental and emotional clutter rivaled the clutter in my neglected home after a year of putting more time into training than cleaning. Ironman New Zealand 2000 was one of my most perfect races in many ways, even though it had the potential to be the worst. What if something happened to my bike on the flight over? How cold would the water be? Would training through the winter temperatures prepare me for the heat of the summer in New Zealand? Did I get enough training in? When I arrived there a week before the race, I found myself doubting my fitness and ability. My amygdala had the potential to make the possible impossible if I had not known how to tiptoe around it. Learning to approach those fears with caution and curiosity changed the outcome of that day profoundly. From developing a spiritual practice for race day, to managing my thoughts and emotions, to performing better than my wildest dreams, it taught me a lot.

All around me, athletes looked in much better shape than I felt. I took a test ride on part of the bike course and felt uneasy. The water was cold, and I had to purchase a long-sleeved wetsuit that I had never raced in before. Easy runs before the event felt hard. How was I going to swim 1.2 miles, bike 112 miles, and then run 26.2 when I struggled with what should have been easy workouts? Fear and doubt had surfaced in my mind and were trying to take over my performance. The perceived pressure I was feeling triggered a fight-or-flight response and I felt adrenaline coursing through my body even when I was trying to sleep. My reactivity was overwhelmingly negative. What if I didn't finish? I am not really an athlete; I'm that overweight, unworthy teenager who was picked last for every team. What will people think of me? Who will listen to me? Who will love me? My amygdala and unharnessed negative emotions clearly had a powerful grip on me, but I had learned healthy and adaptive tools to overcome that control and rewire it to work *for* me rather than against me.

In 1999, the year before Ironman New Zealand, I attended Mark Allen and Brant Secunda's Sport and Spirit workshop. There, I learned so many physical and spiritual lessons that still impact my training, racing, and coaching. My EQ was higher after that workshop. I not only recognized the emotions I felt, but I could manage and shift them to enhance my performance rather than inhibit it. The tools I took away included developing mantras to get me through tough spots, creating ceremonies and making prayer arrows to tap into an energy bigger than myself, and intentionally choosing positive, productive thoughts and emotions over fear and doubt/fight or flight.

I learned how to be in the space of consciousness, to listen to my inner coach rather than my old beliefs. It was a real-time application of tools I had never used before to choose my actions, my thoughts, and my emotions over the course of a long, hard race I had diligently trained for. There was no amygdala hijacking my ability and potential at Ironman New Zealand. Even though there were things I could not control that day, I could control my response to those things.

Race morning, I did a ceremony with the prayer arrow I had learned to make at the workshop. I picked out a quiet, sacred place along the race course and planted the arrow in the sand along the swim course. I knew I would pass it twice in the swim, twice in the bike, and four times in the run. It would be there to remind me to trust myself and powers beyond me.

During the swim, instead of feeling choked by my wetsuit, I focused on the buoyancy it gave me. On the bike, I kept a smile on my face, and when it got hard, I thought about the people in my life who had helped me get to this race; I stayed present rather than thinking about the 26.2 miles I was facing on the run. I had two mantras that carried me those 26.2 miles that reminded me of my purpose and my faith. One was a Huichol Indian song Brant had taught us, and the other was more of a chant: *God's will, God's strength, God's love, I can.* I consider myself more spiritual than religious, so saying "God" for me was unusual, but it worked. The song I sang, and the prayer I said, to the pace of my footfalls on the pavement. Both of these mantras kept me present, positive, and connected to something bigger than myself in a way that I have never experienced before in any of the 11 years of racing prior to that.

Every athlete can learn how to act and how not to react, how to deliberately and consciously choose productive thoughts, how to intentionally generate and cultivate positive emotions to repattern old, performance-inhibiting neurological pathways. Putting these theories into practice in New Zealand in 2000 was the beginning of my realization of the power in those steps and in the power of consciousness as an athlete.

> *A big part of emotional intelligence is learning how to feel an emotion without having to act on it, and how to choose the emotions you want to act on.*

5. Force-feed Success

Rick Hanson talks about carrots and sticks in his book *Buddha's Brain*. We are wired to either approach carrots or avoid sticks. We monitor our environment at all times for experiences that are either pleasant, unpleasant, or neutral. Hanson reminds us that sticks are more powerful than carrots because our brain is built more for avoiding than approaching, and that ability has ensured our survival. Those who learned to avoid danger lived to pass on their DNA. Our brains have an innate ability to detect negative information faster than positive and to store it carefully for future reference. Negative experience, which Hanson describes as "Velcro," has more impact on our lives and feelings than positive experience, and it leaves an enduring memory in your brain. "Your brain has an innate 'negativity bias' that primes you for avoidance." Our positive experience is more like "Teflon" and will slip from our minds unless we develop a way to infuse it into our brains. (Hanson, 2009).

It reminds me of weeds in a garden. You have to spend time and energy keeping your flowers alive, while the weeds seem to persevere even in the toughest of conditions. Droughts, insects, poor soil conditions, and the weeds still manage to pop up, even in the cracks of our driveways after being pulled out for the umpteenth time. Our positive thoughts, like the flowers, need to be tended to on a daily basis, while our negative thoughts, like the weeds, need to be pulled out at the root. Those weeds may always be there just below the surface, but making sure they don't take root and flourish ensures we retrain our garden to be full of flowers instead of weeds.

John was on his college golf team. In his senior year, he was on the 16th hole, down two strokes from the leader and had a putt to shoot an eagle that he could have done in his sleep if there wasn't the pressure of the collegiate championship. His parents, many of his high school and college friends, the press, the coaches, his teammates, and several high-profile golf pros were all there. That shot was the one stroke that would either result in his (perceived) biggest success or biggest failure.

John knew this day would come. He was more than prepared. He had diligently and intentionally practiced success in shots like this over and over in his mind and emotional body. His physical body knew how to do it; he knew he had to get any negative thoughts and emotions out of the way. He had practiced success over and over and over. He had an arsenal of affirmations that prevented the hijack of his amygdala. He knew how to evoke joy in that moment rather than fear, knew what music to listen to to command his confidence, had practiced using his breath to calm his nervous system and find coherence, flow, and the zone, and allow his body to do what it knew how to do.

He had force-fed success into his brain. He had practiced the positive and made it more like Velcro than Teflon. He approached the shot with confidence rather than avoiding it with fear. He had learned how to perceive his situation as positive rather than stressful.

Your amygdala may deliver adrenaline in a sporting situation that includes many spectators and no room for error. Learning to use that adrenaline as a way to enhance performance rather than believe that you will choke is something anyone can learn to do. Your perception of stress is where the stress lies. Being able to shift your perception is where the magic lies.

Without practicing for intense times like John was encountering mentally, given the elevated pressure and stress, either his amygdala would hijack his ability or his higher-thinking prefrontal cortex would "think" it should handle the event. Success does not lie in either of those brain regions. Success is in your body and wired into your neuroanatomy; success will happen if you get out of your own way after force-feeding it into your wiring. Over-fearing or over-thinking anything in sport is not the way to perform. Being positive, in coherence, and in the "autopilot" or striatum of your brain is where performance can be accessed.

The Road Ahead

The structure of our brains really reflects the lives we have lived. The decisions we make, the skills we learn, the choices we make, and the actions we take all end up mapped in the brain like footprints in the sand. Creating new footprints instead of following old ones, one step at a time, is the way to embrace change and to maximize potential. Your brain may be the most adaptable, modifiable, and reprogrammable organ in your body, and it can change for the better or for the worse, depending on how you choose to use it each day. Getting your mind out of the quicksand of your amygdala through practicing these new skills is integral to taking your performance and your life to new levels.

Learning to change your neurology requires beginning with an awareness of your brain's current reality and wiring. A firm grounding and understanding is a powerful springboard to launch from and create the performance and life you desire. You will discover how to make the impossible possible when you hitch your consciousness to your heart's desire rather than let the default programming, unconscious beliefs, and old circuitry of your mind guide your reality.

You can use your life to shape your brain and your dreams will come true.

Cold feet, jealousy, helplessness, hopelessness, nervousness, negativity, overwhelm, sadness, anger, fatigue, not confronting, not asking for help, doubt, second guessing, anxiety, insecurity can lead to

FEAR

which triggers the

AMYGDALA

causing a

RE-ACTION

that

HIJACKS PERFORMANCE.

Confidence, joy, happiness, gratitude, hope, inspiration, awe, serenity, challenge, satisfaction, even smiling can lead to

ACCEPTANCE

which takes the

AMYGDALA

out of the equation, allowing an

ACTION

that

ENHANCES PERFORMANCE.

TOOL #3:
IN-TENTION INSTEAD OF OUT-COME

*Do not dare to live without some clear intention
toward which your living shall be bent. Mean to be
something with all your might.*

—Phillip Brooks

When I first started taking yoga classes, the instructor would have us stand at the top of the mat, close our eyes, and ask us to set an intention for our practice. I wondered what I was supposed to "intend" to do. It was all I could do just to make it through a class without looking like I had no idea *what* I was doing, let alone what I *intended* to do. I may not have had an intention, but I did have a "reason." I was on the mat because I had developed back pain so severe it stopped me, not just from being able to train for an Ironman triathlon I had signed up for, but at times, from even being able to walk. My overtraining and unconsciousness had literally brought me to my knees.

In time, my intention became clear. Short term, it was to recover from injury so I could get back to the training. Now that I look back, however, it was more of an "out-tention," meaning that I was highly focused on a physical *outcome* so I could get back to doing what had put me there in the first place. Each class brought even more awareness, though, as to why I was there, and I soon developed the long-term and more conscious "in-tention" to not just recover from injury and race again, but to use the practice to show up more authentically in sport and in life, and to have a healthier body rather than an injured one.

Intention is the thing that you plan to do or achieve: "an aim or purpose" says Webster's Dictionary. Intention encompasses an ambition, a destination, a design, a direction, an end intended, a fixed purpose, a resolution, a settled determination, a target, and an ultimate purpose. To have and to hold intention means *to have a strong, very personal desire to make something happen in your life.*

Intention is engaging and directing your mind and heart purposefully and your effort steadfastly. When you clarify your desires and shift your thinking and feeling, you can make anything possible. By creating intention, you take responsibility for your future and create a vision for your life. That vision becomes a powerful, heartfelt passion that cannot be seen yet, but can be heard and felt from within.

According to Buddhist teachings, intention is a practice of how you are "being" in the present moment, not necessarily oriented toward a future outcome. Intentions are set based on understanding and aligning your actions and values. They are a grounding for integrity in your life.

In yoga, the term Sankalpa is the word used for intention. From the Sanskrit roots, *san* means a connection to the highest truth, and *kalpa* means vow. It refers to a heartfelt desire or a resolve, and is spoken as an affirmation or declaration in the present tense, starting with "I am." For example, instead of saying "I intend to get strong," you say "I am strong," like a present day, but perhaps deeper version of, an affirmation.

Many times I hear people say, "I never intended for that to happen." But it did happen. If you are not conscious of intention, in sport and in all areas of your life, when you do not *pay attention to your intention*, you may find yourself experiencing an unintentional, or perhaps more to the point, unconscious (un)intentional outcome and reality rather than a conscious one. Your conscious and unconscious intention, your thoughts and beliefs, your emotions and your programming for pain and suffering all create your reality. If you want to create a new reality, *intend* to create something different than the one you are currently experiencing.

When you set that intention, be sure there is not an unintended cost by aiming for a quick outcome instead of steady progress and growth towards it.

For example, exercise is a good thing for us. It not only helps us become fit, it also helps us improve our health. Exercise may help us become more fit than the person who chooses not to exercise, but if we are not intentional and conscious about choosing the right kind and intensity of exercise, we can lose our health by doing more harm than good to our musculoskeletal systems, our immune systems, and sometimes even our mental state. Aiming for outcome, focusing on quantity rather than quality of exercise, training at younger and younger ages, racing more often and longer distances, playing seven games in a single weekend as a young athlete, or applying training programs that focus more on mindless repetition rather than deliberate and intentional practice can all unintentionally make exercise more of a health risk than a health benefit.

Here's the thing: when you set an intention, it is very important to think through the consequences of your choice. Be sure there is not an unintended cost, which there easily can be when you are aiming for *outcome instead of intention and growth*. Frankly, none of us can ultimately control the outcome, but we can instead take *steps toward growth* that can build up and increase the possibility of the positive results of good, healthy intentions.

The only organisms on the planet that incur stress fractures are human beings, race horses, and racing greyhounds. Left to their own devices, the horses and dogs do not develop that injury. We really can be more aware of what our intentions are regarding our health and fitness as opposed to achieving some goal that puts us at risk for injury.

How well I know that to be true. The stress fractures I suffered in my 20s and the low back injury in my 40s were more about my fears and lack of awareness than they were about any intention aimed at improving my overall health and fitness. I had compromised my health for an outcome. I was willing to harm my body with over-training and poor movement patterns to achieve what I thought were important goals, rather than take a step back and protect my body, get out of fear and ego, and intentionally build health and fitness together.

Set Your Intention

Choose your intention carefully and then practice holding your consciousness to it so it becomes the guiding light in your life.

—John Roger

Intention = (a purposeful) Plan + (positively directed) Energy

Intention is not wishful thinking or positive thought and attitude. Intention has an effect like launching an arrow with focus and accuracy at a carefully chosen target. The traditional target has a small bull's eye with concentric rings around it getting larger and larger the further away you move from that center. Intention allows you to make that bull's eye as big in your mind as a whale, and the concentric rings virtually non-existent. When you are able to do that, you will be sure to hit it. When you fill your mind with possibilities and the outcome you desire, there is no room for unintended or undesired outcome. When you feel, see, think, and intend great things as already happening, you can step into them because they are already so. Intentions take energy, effort, commitment, and ownership. I am sure there are many athletes who would like to become world champions or professionals in their sport and have even imagined what it would be like. Just because we want and dream of something, it doesn't automatically follow that it will come to be. We have to be determined to put the energy and resources behind it to make it a true and achievable target.

You create alignment that can make the impossible possible when you set a plan for what you want to achieve. With your purpose in mind, direct your actions with intention and follow through on that plan with commitment. Psychology and spirituality are in agreement that conscious awareness and intention create your reality. Our thoughts and emotions impact everything in our reality from our neural connections to our connection to our world. If you know exactly what you are doing, understand how to do it, and most importantly are conscious of *why* you are doing it, you are far more likely to be successful. You may intend to win a world championship or become a professional in your sport, but do you really understand why you are putting all your energy and resources into those goals?

Are you mindful or mindless? Are you running on a treadmill of unconsciously, neurotically-motivated achievement or finding fulfillment from within?

When you pay attention to your intention, you will carefully determine your thoughts, your words, and your actions—and this inner process will help you keep on course at all times. All your energy will flow in the direction of your goal.

> Are you mindful or mindless? Are you running on a treadmill of unconsciously, neurotically-motivated achievement or finding fulfillment from within?

If your primary intention is acting from a base of healthy thinking and conscious goals, you will most certainly be less likely to damage your body, your mind, or your spirit for the sake of outer achievement. The narrow-focused, potentially harmful, punishing mentality that some of us have brought to sport is misplaced when it costs you your health. That mindset may be a necessary one in rescue work or combat where you have to put your life on the line, but it most certainly is not necessary in sport. What we do as athletes is not a matter of life or death, except maybe to someone's ego—your own or your coach's.

If your intentions do not feel right or good, you are most likely off track. If you are moving toward what brings you pleasure rather than running away from what brings you pain, you are on track. Too often we set goals and intentions based on outcome and about what we want others to think of us or to please them. If you are not enjoying the process or journey, if you are avoiding pain rather than pursuing pleasure, achieving your goals will be bittersweet. The pain you thought you were avoiding will still be following you.

Giving your attention not only to what you are doing, but first understanding the intention behind why you are doing it, will bring you into a higher state of consciousness. This attention and understanding allows you to advance into higher levels of achievement in your sport. The more conscious and deeply-rooted the purpose of your training is, the more invested you will be in it. It may be as simple as the purpose of the exercise you are doing (a shoulder press in the weight room) to the purpose of the training plan (becoming a stronger swimmer) to how it relates to your goals (reducing injury) to how it ties into your life (living the next decades of your life being able to do all the things you love to do).

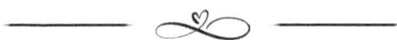

---

*Men are not free when they're doing just
what they like. Men are only free when they're doing
what the deepest self likes. And there is getting
down to the deepest self! It takes some diving.*

—D.H. Lawrence

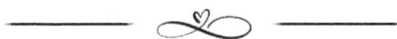

If you don't have a plan for your athletic endeavors, you will never achieve the results you "think" you are able to. The deep roots of intention include planning and structure. It is the framework that your brain thrives on and ultimately will become obedient to. It directs your attention, time, and energy into where you intend to go. Without those roots and framework, your brain is left to its limiting and false beliefs that prevent you from seeing expanded possibilities.

---

*Whether you think you can or
think you can't, you're right.*

—Henry Ford

So many of us talk about what we *can't* do when what we really mean is what we *won't* do. For those of us who look to achieve on the athletic field, it is important to understand what we can't do and how that is different from what we won't do. We may vaguely think that it would be nice to win a gold medal, our age group, or the tournament, but until we truly intend to do it, we have to understand that we are choosing to not put the effort and time and energy into something we say we want to do.

The skill-set you can practice to deepen your intention includes:

1. Saying it
2. Seeing it
3. Feeling it

1. Say Your Intention

Your mind is like a powerful generator constantly putting out thoughts. It cannot really be turned off, but it can be directed or guided consciously. Left to their own devices, thoughts and emotions like doubt and fear build a plan that takes you nowhere near your potential. Those negative thoughts and emotions seep into your performance. Without intention and confidence, you become your own worst enemy. Transforming and directing negative thoughts into hope and possibility are what your mind can do when it creates and directs thoughts with intention.

Take a moment right now and set an intention. Notice how it feels to start to direct your thoughts. Say it out loud. Notice how it feels to put it into words. Does it feel good or is there some hesitation or resistance? Some discomfort is normal, especially if you set a big intention and are not sure yet how you are going to get there.

When you set an intention, add visualization and affirmations of positive thought and then align your feelings and add your heart to the mix. You have the power to create your best outcome.

Louise wanted to make the national team in her sport of flatwater kayak. She set the intention of being on that team. She realized that while there were other women training hard and perhaps faster than her in single boats, she was better in team boats and intended to be in the four-person kayak. She spent time not just on the water training, but also training in her mind. Visualization was something she knew would take her intention to the next level. The negative thought patterns that cluttered her mind were her biggest obstacle. She understood that shifting them to empowering, positive thoughts was the way to train her brain and have it work for her rather than against her.

You can stay connected to an intention with a mantra or affirmation. Mantra, from its Sanskrit roots, means *man*—mind, *tra*—free from. Affirmation, from its Latin roots, means to make steady or strengthen. Both help direct our thoughts and rewire our brains. Imagine that you have to move a heavy boulder that's in your way. If the boulder is too heavy, it will stay in your way and impede any forward progress. But if you have heard of a lever, you can move it with ease. Think of mantras and affirmations like levers. The right tool, with the knowledge of how to use it, makes what you previously thought impossible to be possible. Just like moving a heavy boulder, you can move negative thoughts.

Think of it like a hashtag, something that resonates with you and provides an anchor or motivation when your training gets tough. A mantra could be: "I am strong, lean, and fast." "I am an age group champion." "I am fit from the inside out." "I am powerful, mindful, intentional." "I am the greatest." "I always do my best." "I love being on a team."

Critical thoughts or thoughts that arise out of the exhaustion of the memory of past struggles can erode motivation and performance. Keeping your mind on a mantra can help you stay on track for short- and long-term goals. Your brain gets wired to connect your training with the positive experience of fulfilling your intention. It can also help you stop any negative mental chatter that you might have about your ability or yourself.

Singing is a great way to work thoughts deeper into your psyche. Words with music are better remembered. Singing helps bring calm to our minds and to our bodies and is an easy way to meditate, especially while you are moving. Repeating the same sentences over and over again can free your mind, bring positive energy, and establish a sense of inner ease. One of my clients is recovering from a stroke. She takes part in a music therapy stroke choir at a local hospital, and that therapy has profoundly aided her recovery. When we exercise together, I get her to sing the songs the choir is rehearsing, and she is able to do much more than if she is not singing. Time passes more quickly, it brings a rhythm to her movement, and she is in a much happier state of mind. Like her, I like to sing my affirmations, and I can feel them going deep while doing their important work of uprooting and changing the old negative thoughts and beliefs that hijack my abilities.

If the words that come out of your mouth are positive while the thoughts in your brain are negative, it can feel like you are lying to yourself. Pema Chodron, in her book *Start Where You Are,* tells us, "Affirmations are like screaming that you're okay in order to overcome the whisper that you are not." (Chodron, 2001). Perhaps those whispers uncovered will help you reveal your fears and false beliefs and help you be brave enough to confront them. You can be scared and still intend to do your best.

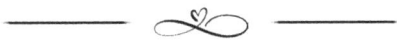

*Music gives a soul to the universe, wings to the
mind, flight to the imagination, life to everything.*

—Plato

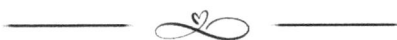

LABEL	
BAD	GOOD
NEGATIVE	POSITIVE
AMYGDALA/STRESS/NO CHANGE	CORTEX/EASE/CHANGE

2. See Your Intention

Every minute of every day, we visualize using our powerful imaginations to create certain things in our lives. You may not even be aware of it on a conscious level, but just think about it for a minute and understand how every morning you wake up and you see yourself navigating your way through your day. If you are dreading an early track workout, you are already unconsciously creating your reality. You unconsciously use your imagination in a negative way rather than for positive growth.

Think of how many times your fear of losing or underperforming came true. Fear and doubt will always trickle down into performance, and you created that reality with your powerful imagination and visualization. Creating a mental image of what you intend to happen or to feel has a powerful effect on reality. Seeing yourself succeed or perform and feel in a positive way aligned with your conscious intentions creates the reality you intend.

Despite the fact that visualization and meditation have been around for millennia, it hasn't been that long in recent history that using visualization or imagery at elite levels was talked about. Research has since shown that intending to see success triggers responses from the autonomic nervous system and creates neural patterns in your brain that improve athletic performance at all levels, from novices to elites. Even five minutes of imagery can make a significant difference in performance. You can see success in your mind and feel it in your body long before you actually perform it in the real world.

Many elite athletes will tell you they train their physical bodies in practice and in competition, and they also train their bodies *in their minds* using imagery. Awareness increases, along with confidence. They visualize and imagine what they intend to happen, and they often do it in great detail. Creating a mental image of what you intend to happen and stepping into how you intend to feel will have a powerful effect on what really happens. Visualization can be used for training sessions and for competition. Seeing and feeling yourself succeed in the way you intend has immense power. Our emotional states and perceptions play the dominant role in creating a coherent physiological state, preparing us for optimal performance.

In 1984, when 235 Canadian Olympic athletes were preparing for the Games in Los Angeles, they were surveyed about their training. Almost all—99 percent of them—used imagery (Orlick, 1988). Timothy Gallowey, author of *The Inner Game of Tennis* tells us, "Athletic improvement without the development of mental skills (such as visualization) is impossible." (Gallowey, 1997)

Visualizing is like being able to travel into the future with your senses and emotions, lay down a blueprint or imprint of success while you are there, and bring it back to the present moment. It can be a very powerful tool in your daily life, using the same part of your brain consciously without having the body actually perform. Your mind just "thinks" that it is. Before you can actually execute success with your body, your thoughts, senses, and emotions have a neurological imprint, so to speak, of that success. It is the process of creating a mental image or intention of what you want to happen and feel in reality. Visualizing can include more than just mental images. You can create kinesthetic sensations inside and out, along with auditory sounds that inspire you, in your mind. You can rehearse saying, seeing, feeling, and hearing the outcome you desire.

The reason imagery works is that your brain itself is not smart. It can be tricked—or in this case, trained. As far as your brain is concerned, what you imagine actually happens and your body believes it, too. When your eyes are closed, your brain does not know where it is. If you are imagining being at your favorite golf course successfully finishing 18 holes eight under par, your brain and body believe you. You can tell it with guided imagery, visualization, daydreaming, or imagining. Chemically, it does not know the difference between what you are experiencing in real time and what you are using your consciousness to imagine. When you visualize a skill, the same motor and sensory programs that are involved in actually doing it will be engaged. Cognitive processes in the brain, including perception, memory, and attention, are also affected. Every thought leaves a physical signature. So in visualizing the perfect execution of a skill, a game, or a race, you map out with intention that signature in your brain and subsequently in your body. Physical and psychological reactions in pressure situations can be improved by consciously and deliberately practicing visualization techniques. They can result in a very vivid experience where you have far more control over a successful performance and belief in yourself.

Set a very specific goal for yourself, imagine achieving your goal, see yourself achieving your goal, and then see and feel all of the details with all of your senses.

———— ✧ ————

Imagination is more important than science.

—Albert Einstein

———— ✧ ————

You can experience real change when you are conscious of who you are, when your mind and body are in alignment, and when you come to fully realize your state of being as an observer of yourself, your thoughts, and your feelings. When you observe and choose a new outcome with a new mind, you can implement the power of intention.

When you have an intentional thought with the catalyst of an intentional emotion, you are using the power of those frequencies and forces to use thoughts, beliefs, and feelings to emit and broadcast the energy of winning and success.

3. Feel Your Intention

Powerful Intention = Intentional Thought + Elevated Emotion

In my experience, everything is energy. I believe that negative thoughts and feelings have a low frequency. Positive thoughts and feelings have a high frequency. Beliefs are the filter of the thousands of random thoughts and feelings that go through our minds and bodies on a daily basis. If it is just a fantasy that you will achieve success, if you don't really believe it, then it is not really possible for you to succeed. When your thoughts and feelings are not consistent with your beliefs, then the impossible blocks what is possible. The greatest success happens when an athlete sets an intention, visualizes and feels it in detail, and believes in this new "self" achieving that goal.

Emotions are magnetic; thoughts are electric. The electrical field of the heart is about 60 times greater in amplitude than the brain, and the magnetic component of the heart is 5,000 times stronger than that produced by the brain. (McCraty, 2003).

So positive thoughts, then are not nearly as powerful as positive emotions. Intention point is the meeting ground between your mind and your heart. When you rewire and reprogram your heart, there is more power in your intention. The Fifth Step in becoming conscious is intentional generation of a positive state of physiological coherence. You know that emotion will trump logic: the practice of generating positive emotions intentionally will help to physiologically and psychologically achieve a powerful intention for each and every workout, race, performance, practice, game, or match. Imagine being able to dial up your wattage from the inside out. You might believe that increasing your power on your bike helps you improve; now, imagine dialing up the power on your thoughts and emotions and intentions.

The use of power versus force is an important concept in sport, intention, and consciousness. The word "power" is rooted in the old French *pouvoir*: to be able, and Latin *potus*: powerful. (Etymology Dictionary, 2021). It is a combination of forces and movement, the ability to act or produce a desired effect. Force, on the other hand, is rooted in old French *forcer*: conquer by violence, exert force upon. (Etymology Dictionary, 2021). It is a push or pull upon an object resulting from the object's interaction with another object. We tend to use force, stress, or resistance instead of power to move our bodies or play our sport. When you force your training, based on ego, false beliefs, or fear towards where you think you need to go, it can cause more pushing against. It isn't until you stop pushing that any real allowing of what you want can take place, that you can find your own power. Forcing something implies you want something outside of yourself to change, rather than you making a change in yourself. Force is coercion. Power is allowing.

David Hawkins, MD, Ph.D. tells us in his book *Power vs Force*, that if you can raise your consciousness to levels of power rather than force, you will become awake and aware and your life will most certainly never be the same. He tells us that impossible becomes possible when we surrender to the essence of life and move beyond the "apparent" limit of our abilities. (Hawkins, 2013).

I advise all my athletes to set a goal; a powerful intention based on intentional thought and positive emotion with regards to their race season and prioritize their races. Then I advise them to detach from the outcome. It is good to have goals and aspirations, but it is best to use a compass to guide your journey rather than fix your sights on a destination, a finish line. Understand that the return on your investment of time and energy may not be what you expect. Who amongst us has not found ourselves working so hard towards a desired outcome but no matter how hard we worked, it just didn't pay off like we expected it to? We can only act with good intentions and then let go and trust that whatever the outcome is, it is the right one. If you work hard and then let go of your outcome, you might find an unexpected return on that investment. I am finding that the best things in my life have come not when I have pushed (forced), but when I have stepped into my power (allowed) and learned to let go.

Creating intention is powerful. It is the beginning of something bigger, something important you want in your life. You get to decide what that is and how to focus on it to the best of your abilities. It is a vision for your sport and your life. That vision is an energy in your heart, full of power and passion that you may not be able to see right now, but it can be felt and heard deep inside you. *By creating intention, you are acknowledging you want something to change in your life and you are taking responsibility for finding the solution.* It may be uncomfortable and you may feel resistance, and that is where growth happens. When you learn to banish doubt and trust in your powerful and passionate feelings, you clear a path for the power of your intention to flow through.

What can you do?

Intentional thought + elevated emotion = powerful intention aligned with beliefs and actions taken

- Make a list of intentions and align yourself with them.
- Align yourself with people, opportunities, mentors, and coaches who are positive and support your intention.

- Clear out anything that is not in alignment with your intention—thoughts, beliefs, behaviors, emotions, people—and replace it consciously with everything that does.
- Deliberately practice visualizing and feeling your intention.
- Be grateful and responsible. Be accountable for yourself and your actions.
- Take one action every day in the direction of your intention. Pattern your behavior in the direction of your desire.
- Develop your own mantras and affirmations.
- Instruct your body with feelings to change its chemistry so that the body understands what the mind intellectually knows.
- Neurologically and chemically condition the body to do as well as the conscious mind believes it can: the teaching becomes innate; the result is mastery.

THOUGHTS	EMOTIONS	ACTIONS	BELIEFS
electric	magnetic	conscious	changeable
INTENTIONAL	ELEVATED	DELIBERATE	ALIGNED

―――――――― ✌◯ ――――――――

You are your deepest DESIRES
As is your desire, so is your INTENTION
As is your intention, so is your WILL
As is your will, so is your DEED
As is your deed, so is your DESTINY

—The Upanishads

―――――――― ✌◯ ――――――――

TOOL #4:
THE POWER OF MEDITATION

———— ❧ ————

Meditation brings wisdom; lack of meditation leaves ignorance. Know well what leads you forward and what holds you back, and choose the path that leads to wisdom.

—Buddha

———— ❧ ————

Imagine how it would feel to step up to the starting line or onto the field or the court with a smile on your face, feeling confident and calm, having clarity, focused only on the task at hand, being in control of your emotions, having an inner state of relaxed awareness, *and experiencing no anxiety about the outcome?*

> Meditation isn't controlling your thoughts and emotions; it is stopping your thoughts and emotions from controlling you.

You would feel totally absorbed in what you were doing. Time would slow down. You would feel joy. Your performance would feel effortless and exceed your expectations.

If you have not experienced that kind of confidence and control, your mind is most likely not as well trained as your body. Confidence and control are the performance-enhancing drugs of champions. Learning to train your brain and untangle your thoughts, to focus your attention and intention, are critical skills to elevate you to peak performance. The reality may be that it is not what more our bodies are capable of, but what more our minds can do to take our bodies to the next level of capability. *Meditation isn't controlling your thoughts and emotions; it is stopping your thoughts and emotions from controlling you.*

Just as any skill you require to excel in your sport needs to be practiced, so does meditation. Expecting to have a clear mind over which you are in full control the moment you sit down to meditate is like expecting to be able to run a four-minute mile your first time on the track. A mind that is not under control is more likely to make mistakes, mistakes that could prevent you from performing your best. Your mind, like your body, must be trained with deliberate, intentional practice. Meditation is working with your thoughts. It teaches you to clear your mind of thoughts that sabotage performance and consciously choose those that enhance it. Some say that sport is up to 90 percent mental, yet we spend 90 percent of our time, money, and effort on physical and technical training, and not on mental training. In Step Two, we looked at practicing with an open or beginner's mind; meditation will help you open and clear your mind so new insights and answers can arise.

What Can Meditation Do For You?

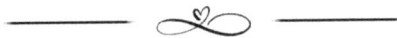

———— ✌✌ ————

It's through our meditation practice that we can enter the subconscious and change our unwanted programs. Think of the subconscious as the brain's operating system. By dropping into the operating system of the brain, we can alter habits, behaviors, and remove emotional scars. If you're not trying to change anything, you can simply open yourself up to receiving unknown possibilities and create something new.

—Dr. Joe Dispenza

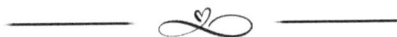

———— ✌✌ ————

Meditation offers you the potential to gain mastery of your mind by restructuring your brain. By mastering your mind, you have the power to master your emotions, your thoughts, and your performance.

In the book *Altered Traits*, the authors tell us: "The original aim, (of meditation) embraced still in some circles to this day, focuses on a deep exploration of the mind toward a profound alteration of our very being." They speak to the original deep path with a spiritual focus, and the wide paths of meditation that have developed that leave behind some of the original, ancient practices. If you want to go deep, you may find qualities not necessarily specific to your sport, but will cultivate traits such as selflessness, equanimity, compassion, and a loving presence. (Goleman, Davidson, 2017). Not only can meditation give power to your mind, it can also open your heart.

Research shows that neuroanatomical changes happen at cortical and subcortical levels where the areas of perception and regulation of emotions lie. (D'Arista, Egiziano, Gardi, Petrosino, Vatti et al, 2014). Meditation is a simple way to work with the power of your mind to develop new areas of your brain and to realize a huge return on the investment you make. Not only can meditation develop new areas of your brain like the hippocampus that assists in learning, memory, and emotional regulation, it can also help shrink your amygdala. As discussed in Tool #2, being able to respond rather than react can immensely enhance performance.

Imagine that your mind is like a big house you have been living in for years and in it are doors you have never opened. All the familiar doors are the mind's habitual ways of thinking and responding unconsciously and habitually. You may not have even known other doors were there. Through meditation you can find and open them, and in doing so, expand your world and your ability to understand and respond to the reality of that new world.

The good news is that while meditation offers profoundly positive results, as a practice, it is actually quite simple. There really isn't a wrong or right way to meditate or any big mystery about it. Just as there are many different ways to swing a golf club, there are different meditation techniques that will work best for you.

The most common vehicle you can use to untangle yourself from jumpy, wild, emotion-based thoughts to help you meditate is to focus on your breath. Since the mind and the breath work in tandem, when you bring your breath into conscious control, you can use it to slow down the chatter of your mind and body that so often interferes with performance. Focusing on the inhale, the exhale, and the space in between gives the brain an anchor to hold onto and invites the mind to quiet and calm.

Learning to find clarity, strength, courage, and the elusive zone will become easier when you learn to respond to situations from a calm and grounded place rather than reacting to them from a stressed and anxious place. Finding a way to have a calm and uncluttered mind is really all you need to do. An unfocused, cluttered mind coupled with short, shallow breath creates a tense, confused body. A clear directive from an uncluttered mind and deep, controlled breath creates a calm, confident body where anything becomes possible.

This focused breathing oxygenates our brains, and over time, focusing on that slower rhythm helps us understand ourselves and the world that we race through. Taking time to "be," to simply breathe, experiencing the most basic mechanism of survival, gives us an opportunity to open up our awareness and tap into our intuition. In that focus and space, you can learn to recognize thought patterns, belief systems, and the emotions associated with them that may be inhibiting your performance, and more importantly, guide you towards your true nature.

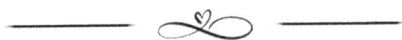

———— ⚬ ————

If the ocean can calm itself, so can you.
We are both salt water mixed with air.

—Nayyirah Waheed

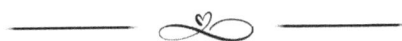

———— ⚬ ————

I have mentioned many times in this book that we most often don't make changes until it's too painful not to change. Not only that, you can't change what you don't notice. Meditation and breath give you the opportunity to notice and the power to change those old beliefs, thoughts, and emotional responses that are not serving you and most likely interfering with your athletic potential.

Your ability to recognize what is going through your mind and control is a core strength you can build. Meditation may be the first opportunity in your life for you to realize that a thought or emotion you have is not your only version of reality; you can focus on something else, like your breathing, and just let that thought or emotion simply pass by. You can then create your own version of the reality you want to live in.

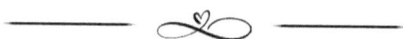

To breathe fully is to live fully, to manifest the full range of power of our inborn potential for vitality in everything that we sense, feel, think, and do.

—The Tao of Natural Breathing

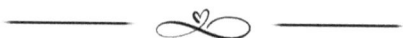

Meditation and Consciousness

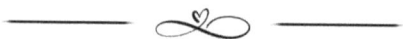

Meditation is the dissolution of thoughts in external awareness or pure consciousness.

—Sivananda

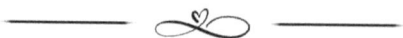

Meditation is a tool you can use to train your mind and become more conscious as an athlete. In essence, it is a state of pure consciousness without thought. It is a mental practice that develops intelligence and sharpens the mind. If you haven't tried it yet, be prepared to take your game to a whole new level. You may have tried meditation sitting on a floor or cushion in some pretzel-like position that was incredibly uncomfortable with your tight hips, closed your eyes, tried to breathe and stop your thoughts, all the while feeling frustrated with the "spoiled child" or "monkey mind" running wild in your head even more than it usually does.

Imagine the thoughts in your mind as drunken monkeys—loud, obnoxious, and rambunctious—or as a spoiled child that throws temper tantrums, is never satisfied, expects your full attention and most often ignores you. Your mind is housing dozens of drunken monkeys or spoiled children all looking for your attention. The children and monkeys of negative emotions like fear and anxiety tend to demand a lot of our awareness. You may be laughing as you recognize that spoiled child and drunken monkey running around in your own mind, but I can guarantee you they do nothing to enhance your performance.

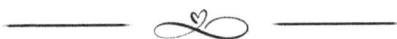

--------- ❧ ---------

Don't let anyone rent a space in your head
unless they are a good tenant.

—Michael Singer

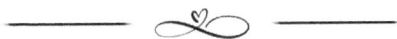

--------- ❧ ---------

Just as physical exercise conditions the body, conscious cognitive training rewires the mind. If you learn to focus on the present moment, reduce distraction and stress, choose your thoughts and emotions, and strengthen the mind-body connection, you will unlock a new level of competition. Consider meditation as the strengthening of your mind the way weightlifting strengthens your body. Meditation is a powerful way to shift out of deeply held mindsets and beliefs that may be holding you back from your full potential. Learning to change your mindset will allow you to more quickly realize the results you desire physically.

Meditation is a way to heightened consciousness and timelessness. You may not sit and chant, but you can learn to do it in the flow of sport. Increasing your awareness rather than your effort is where moments become magical, where there is all the time in your world to do incredible things—run faster, jump higher, think clearer—by moving into increased consciousness.

As an athlete, I have preferred to practice what I like to refer to as *moving meditation,* although I have recently been developing a practice of stillness (which is much harder than I thought it would be). It seems to take more effort not to move than to move. Many of us as athletes find that when our bodies are fully engaged and our minds are focused on the task at hand, our monkey mind doesn't run around so much. Sport often requires 100 percent of your attention where you are completely in the present, focused or "meditating" on exactly what is required of you in that moment. That kind of focus requires a detachment from the monkey mind.

Merriam Webster defines meditation as engaging "in contemplation or reflection, to focus on one's thoughts, to reflect or ponder over, and to plan or project in the mind: intend, purpose." (Merriam Webster, 2023).

The Tibetan word for meditation is *gom,* which can be translated as "to become familiar with." (Ripoche, 2016). It implies the ability to train the mind to become familiar with beneficial states of consciousness such as concentration, correct understanding, perseverance, patience, and humility. Not only can our conscious thoughts be brought under control, but also our emotions and "unconsciousness," as they are all based on concepts which can be changed.

If your goal is to become more conscious as an athlete, meditation is a way to alter your level and state of awareness. It is a consciousness-changing technique that has many benefits for you as an athlete regarding both your performance and your overall health. It will increase your awareness and sharpen your ability to focus your attention. It has been practiced for thousands of years, across virtually every religion and culture, and there are many different ways to practice it.

There are two main types of meditation. One teaches you how to focus on a single thing and tune everything else out around you. The other teaches you how to reduce stress and enhance cognition. These are good skills to have if you want to improve as an athlete.

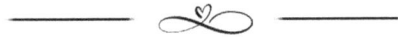

———— ⚮ ————

The goal of meditation is NOT to get rid of thoughts or emotions. The goal is to become more aware of thoughts and emotions and to learn how to move through them without getting stuck.

—Dr. P. Goldin

———— ⚮ ————

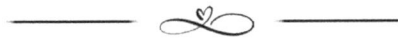

Your consciousness is like a stream flowing through your mind. Recall John Locke's definition of consciousness: "...the perception of what passes in a man's own mind." It runs all day long, whether you realize it or not, and it will shift and change smoothly and effortlessly as the terrain and the environment it navigates shifts. What flows through your mind sculpts your brain. Your mind is simply information that is being moved by your nervous system like blood is moved by the heart; it is your brain in action. When you learn to make your brain work differently, you change your mind.

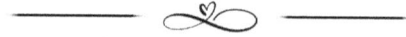

Meditation makes the entire nervous system go into a field of coherence.

—Deepak Chopra

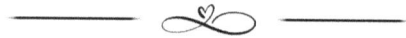

Meditation and the Brain

Our minds wander naturally, somewhere between 30 and 70 percent, depending on what you are doing and how focused you are. At times, it is beneficial for you to allow that wandering. It can lead to new and innovative ideas. You can use your brain to change your mind and how it flows to serve you better by bringing it into your conscious awareness. Thought, unconscious and unguarded, can harm your performance, especially if it wanders into negative thoughts rather than the task at hand.

Meditation is a way to observe that stream, work your brain differently, reduce the wandering and direct its course while shifting how you perceive and respond to the environment around you. What you pay attention to is a decision you can make rather than having what you pay attention to be decided by shifts in your environment. I am reminded of the movie *Up,* where the golden retriever, Dug, who is smart and able to converse with human beings, always runs the risk of being distracted by a squirrel that enters his awareness. In the middle of a conversation, his brain yells, "Squirrel!" and off he goes in pursuit of it. Our thoughts and perceptions can distract us from what we are focused on at any given moment if we unconsciously allow them to.

Our ability to choose what we pay attention to has to do with not only being able to sharpen our focus, but also to be able to tune out distractions. When you increase your focus, the brain works to synchronize activity in different regions, like getting on the same frequency so communication is open. When you tune out distractions, your brain has to actively suppress what is irrelevant.

Mindfulness meditation trains the prefrontal cortex of your brain, which is responsible for executive function. It is the conductor of your brain, coordinating and guiding functions of other areas. In terms of enhancing sport, it is a key area to develop because it is associated with attention, distraction, cognition, arousal, decision-making, insight, and emotion. The brain of an athlete demands high-speed decision-making, the ability to visualize, to regulate emotions, and to focus along with high awareness, quick reaction time, spatial thinking, and reasoning. Small changes in your mind become big changes in your brain.

The prefrontal cortex is also where our calm but alert mind resides. Being able to stay in the calm and confident cortex, not in the fight or flight of your amygdala, decreases stress that could negatively impact performance. Reducing stress creates a more resilient mind. Training our prefrontal cortex also activates the insular cortex that allows us to experience a heightened awareness of our bodies and improve mind-body communication.

The same way we have drunken monkeys and spoiled children running through our minds, we have a logical, rational "human" mind (prefrontal cortex) and an irrational, emotional, "chimp" mind (amygdala). Dr. Steve Peters, in his book *The Chimp Paradox*, explains how emotions often dictate without our conscious permission and create havoc in our performance and our lives. (Peters, 2013). Our chimp hijacks our minds unless we learn how to harness it and use it only when necessary.

When you find yourself in the right regions of your brain, when you have the right balance between your nervous systems, when you consciously choose the thoughts and emotions that use your neurology to enhance your performance, you have harnessed a new power and limitless potential.

*Through meditation and by giving full attention
to one thing at a time, we can learn to direct
attention where we choose.*

—Eknath Easwaran

Benefits of Meditation for Athletes

*It is easier to develop the mind through meditation
than it is just through athletic practice. If you put
the two together, it will be unbelievable.*

—Frederick Lenz

Meditation reduces stress by changing the way our nervous system responds to what it perceives as stress. Too much stress not only affects your performance, it also affects your well-being. Studies have shown how our sympathetic nervous system stress hormones negatively affect our bodies and brains and how meditation helps reduce those hormones. Staying calm and focused under pressure, anchored to the present moment with higher self-confidence and increased concentration, can only enhance performance.

Meditation helps you learn to balance your emotional quotient. Not being swayed off course by negative emotions is one of the keys to success. Becoming aware of those emotions is an important step. Missing a putt in your golf game, a basket in your basketball game, a serve in your volleyball game doesn't mean that error must be brought into the rest of your game. Breath and meditation are directly linked to your emotions and your ability to control and choose them. They help us become mentally stronger and give us a say over whether or not we allow those emotions that inhibit our performance. Competitive minds often live on a roller coaster ride of emotions. Learning to meditate teaches you to stabilize your mood rather than have it control you and your performance.

Meditation helps you stay in the present moment with a calm mind and clear thought. Often our minds swing between the future and the past, locking us into a stress response, keeping us from the current flow of events.

"I don't want to lose to this team again."

"Last time I really messed up my routine."

Thoughts like that take you out of the present and predict a negative outcome before it has even happened. If you are not in the "current flow" of awareness, you are unconsciously operating in the "under-current of chaos" that will sabotage your performance no matter how highly skilled you might be physically.

A mind that is habituated and falls into grooves with no room for change limits us. Meditation gives you greater mental awareness, which helps you adapt and learn by weakening existing connections between neurons that only process information habitually based on your previous experiences and perceptions. You may learn new techniques with more ease and less effort and adapt to new situations and environments without feeling stressed. You can develop the ability to manipulate and maintain several objects of attention by increasing the working memory capacity of your brain.

Meditation teaches your mind to stay focused and find clarity in chaos. It allows the brain to think quicker, be more intuitive, and dismiss fear. When you are on the free throw line unable to focus, you will most likely miss your shot. Every athlete, no matter what sport, can benefit from stronger focus skills. Optimal mind-body integration and coordination ensure success under pressure.

Meditation teaches you how to cope with pressure. You learn to reduce feelings of anxiety and nervousness as pressure mounts.

Did you ever experience a time in your athletic life where you stepped up to a bigger venue and "should" have performed or placed better, but you "choked" because you could not control your stress? Choking, by definition, is not being able to breathe, or the sensation of something stuck in your throat. The intense visceral response we have in sport to stress we cannot deal with is aptly named. When breath allows your mind to work effortlessly with your body at peak ability, the combination results in peak levels of performance. You will have more precision in your actions when the mind and body are cooperating rather than competing.

Meditation studies have shown that the nervous system actually begins responding differently to stressful situations: creativity flows more freely and new solutions begin to emerge. (Bauer, 2022). Instead of reacting from fear, you act from centered calm. Remember that the amygdala can hijack your performance. Meditation helps you learn how to calm it, even when you are not meditating. When we lose games, perform below our ability, or fail miserably, it's hard not to obsess about those perceived negative experiences and then be able to bounce back. A quiet mind stops thought, which stops resistance and gives you access into the state of allowing.

Meditation has also been shown to increase the quality of our sleep and reduce recovery time from training, racing, and injury. Cortisol levels and post-workout perceived pain can be significantly reduced by meditating for a few minutes post-workout to enhance those aspects of recovery. It deepens relaxation and improves overall well-being. If you are sick, you are on the sidelines. A night of lost sleep could lose a championship. By boosting our immune system and resiliency, we can function and perform at higher levels.

In addition, meditation helps remove our blind spots. Remember Step #3, where you took your inventory? There were blind spots and beliefs outside of your awareness that may have had a choke hold on you, limiting your performance, or were abilities waiting to surface and take you to new heights. Regardless of helping or hindering performance, the blind spots and beliefs are obstacles. Meditation is a way to help bring those obstacles to light, along with the potential power they have to enhance performance or stop inhibiting it.

How to Meditate

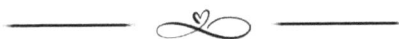

*If you want to find God, hang out in
the space between your thoughts.*

—Alan Cohen

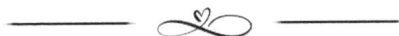

Meditation began as a way to find spiritual enlightenment, a way to understand self and the world in a deep and transforming way, an awakening. Today, it is gaining ground as a way to enhance performance in athletes and top executives, a technique to reduce stress, and a practice to accelerate and promote healing. We now know there are countless benefits of meditation for our brains, bodies, immune systems, nervous systems, intelligence, emotions, and stress levels.

In the Buddhist tradition, meditation is a word like sport is to us. It refers to a multitude of activities, not just one. It may be difficult for you to sit on a cushion with an empty mind for 45 minutes, but you may be able to sit where you are right now and bring your consciousness to your breath. Regardless of what kind of mindfulness and meditation makes sense to you, there is no way to be successful without first passing through the gate of breathing. You can start a deliberate meditation practice to manage your thoughts and feelings, change your neurology and belief systems, and enhance your performance with physical and mental gains.

---

*Like riding a bike or playing tennis, what I want
you to understand is relaxing the body yet staying
conscious is just a skill to develop (there's a reason
why we call meditation a practice). When you
can completely relax your body and remain
conscious, this is the realm where the unknown
and the mystical happens.*

—Dr. Joe Dispenza

Meditation 101

1. Sit or lie comfortably. Move gently if you prefer.
2. Close your eyes or soften your focus.
3. Allow your breath to happen naturally.
4. Focus your attention on the breath and on how the body responds to each inhalation, exhalation, and the pause between. Notice the subtle movement of your body as you breathe. Observe your chest, back, shoulders, rib cage, and belly. Simply notice and focus your attention on your breath without controlling its pace or intensity.
5. Detach from thoughts and the idea of not doing it right. If your mind wanders, simply observe it and return your focus back to your breath.
6. Use a mantra or a single word if you find it useful to anchor you.
7. Use a video or audio to guide you if you find it easier to begin with.

Maintain the meditation practice for two or three minutes to start, and then progress with longer periods as you are ready.

Meditation Technology

There is no scientific study more vital to man than the study of his own brain. Our entire view of the universe depends on it.

—Francis Crick

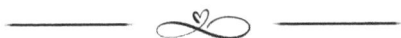

I use Muse, a meditation technology which uses the validated science of real-time electroencephalogram (EEG) technology that has delivered the opportunity to support and improve brain health and performance. The brain-sensing headband makes the practice of meditation more quantifiable and tangible and allows you to see in real time which brain wave you are in. As I mentioned, my meditation practice in stillness needs work. Muse encourages me to practice every day, tracks my progress, and even reminds me that there are benefits whether I record time in calm, active, or neutral brain activity. It has most certainly helped me clear my cluttered mind, be more mindful and present, breathe, and find more ease and less effort in sport and in life.

In his book, *The Brain Always Wins*, Dr. John Sullivan explains why the brain matters in sport and how it impacts our performance and our health. Learning to use our brain to serve us rather than unconsciously allowing it to have power over us means we can improve our performance through consciously managing our minds and subsequently changing the structure of our brain.

Muse technology has made the process of meditation practice more scientific, tangible, and, in turn, approachable. The information gained and "gamified" allows the end user and sport scientist to guide and measure not only improvement but protection of brain health. Thus, the contemplative traditions of meditation aiming to bring the practitioner closer to self-actualization and enlightenment can do so—and that fits nicely with the goals of the sport environment which are based in health and performance, and which are also contemporary conceptualizations of advancing human potential. (Sullivan and Parker, 2016).

There are many meditation apps you can use to help guide you. My personal favorite is Insight Timer, and you can get it for free. It is currently home to over 19 million meditators, has 130,000 free guided meditations, music tracks, and courses, and features over 17,000 teachers. Insight Timer tells us the app is the largest conscious classroom in the world. You can select by time for short or long meditations and see your stats and milestones as your progress is tracked. The guided meditations and talks are led by the world's best meditation and mindfulness experts. Neuroscientists, psychologists, and teachers from Ivy League schools share their insights. Music from world-renowned artists will soothe and stimulate your heart, mind, and brain. Insight Timer is great for both beginners and experienced practitioners.

When you understand that learning to meditate doesn't require moving to the Himalayas, and you know why you are doing it, you can use it to move through all Five Steps to Consciousness very quickly. Your awareness and internal focus will increase, your mind, and heart will be more open, you will come to understand yourself better, and you will deliberately and intentionally tap into your abilities physiologically and psychologically.

Take that breath I discussed in Chapter 2 and use it as a ramp to start the changes you can make from the inside out.

TOOL #5:
THE POWER OF CHANGE

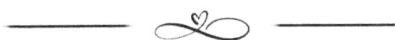

How strange that the nature of life is change,
yet the nature of human beings is to resist change.

—Elizabeth Lesser

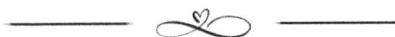

In choosing to read this book, you are already practicing the skill of deliberate change. You can't change what you don't notice. By making the choices to come into consciousness and awareness, to turn your focus inward to figure out where you are headed and why you are headed there, you have noticed what needs to be changed.

It's much easier to quantify the results of your sport than it is to measure "inner" success. Regardless, if you want a life that is full and fulfilling, you must develop a sense of who you are, look to understand why you do what you do, and how your thoughts, feelings, and beliefs encourage, define, and represent you in your sport and in your life. Whether you are looking to simply change your technique in the pool, take your game to a new level of performance, look at other ways to improve besides training harder, or perhaps more profoundly, change the quality of yourself and your life, you have begun to wake up and take the steps outlined earlier in the book.

The results you so ardently want to realize, manifest, and achieve are well within the realm of possibility. As I've mentioned before, I believe anything is possible. Impossible becomes possible when you develop these new skills. But you must be willing and able to step away from old, well-worn, circular, and most often unconscious paths that keep you stuck and make change seem impossible. It is in the exploring of untried paths beyond those old familiar ones where change can really happen and results become possible.

This is not about changing who you are, but it is about becoming aware of the positive and negative thoughts, ideas, beliefs, emotions, and behaviors so you are in conscious control of them. It's about learning to recognize your reactions and understand why you feel that way. Our brains know how to take short cuts and make behaviors as automatic as possible. That frees our minds up for potentially more important matters. More often than not, change is about changing what we "want," not what we "do". If you want to eat healthier, but burgers and fries are your comfort foods, replacing them with broccoli and carrots is like trying to fix a flat tire on your bike by getting new handlebars. You don't need a new diet, you need an alternative way to feel comfort.

So how do you make those changes?

Let's look at six ways to begin with.

1. Consciously decide and choose to change
2. Work hard, be patient, take baby steps
3. Keep an open heart and mind
4. Practice undoing, letting go, and lose your mind
5. Rewire mental and emotional neural circuitry
6. Choose your emotions and follow them into a conscious future

1. Consciously Decide and Choose to Change

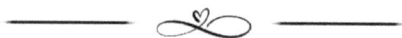

Things do not change; we change.

—Henry David Thoreau

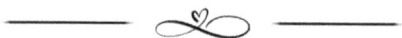

Change means to make or become different, to replace something with another, to make a shift, to undergo a modification or transformation. It can happen when you meet limited circumstances with unlimited thoughts. Anything is possible if you have the capacity and willingness to change.

Peter Jensen, a sport psychologist, in his book *Ignite the Third Factor*, borrows a concept from one of his teachers, Kazimierz Danowski, that he saw as important in the development and growth of athletes as people. The first two factors he considers are nature and nurture. They establish the template of our physical and mental bodies along with the social and physical aspects of our lives that help shape us. He speaks to a third factor, a factor of choice, which allows us to transcend our parents and our experiences to change and become a highly functioning athlete and person. (Jensen, 2011).

That third factor of choice allows you to uncover and display what you possess. He describes unsuccessful programs about pushing change. He agrees with the Buddhists who tell us, "Don't push the river. It will move at its own pace." We can move in the direction that the water flows, or we can swim hard against it. There is more success in moving with the flow than exhausting ourselves trying to move against it. Igniting choice is about being drawn toward, pulled, or being grounded in the direction you are moving towards. You choose to consciously move towards growth rather than being pushed or chased towards something you are not ready for or do not want.

> When you don't *force* change but *choose* it, you redefine possibility.

When you don't *force* change, but *choose* it, you redefine possibility.

Change is inevitable in life and in sport. There is no way around it. Most of us are convinced that change is "hard." And perhaps it is if it is being forced. But the reality is that we are an adaptable organism designed to change in order to survive. Adaptation is the rule of human existence. Hard just means it takes effort and commitment,

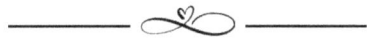

characteristics that all athletes possess. There are many changes in life that are not under our control, but there are some we can deliberately and intentionally change: our behaviors, thoughts, feelings, and habits.

The Ancient Greeks spoke of a philosophical conundrum, the "paradox of the heap." In 400 B.C., they asked the question: At what point do single grains of sand become a heap of sand? One, two, or 20 grains are certainly not, but when you add one grain at a time, there is an eventual shifting point where the "heap" is formed. The question is, when does that happen? The point at which things change is more often a figment of our imagination (what we believe) than when it actually does happen.

I have said many times that we never make a change until it's too painful not to. Obstacles to change include negativity, distraction, disinterest, and even active resistance. Complacency and inertia can also stop new ideas and limit potential. The same way you can shift your behaviors into change, into a new heap, you can slowly shift out of the old heap of behaviors you built that have become too painful to keep repeating. We unconsciously choose the familiarity of the status quo over the fear of the unknown, even when the status quo may no longer be serving us.

When you deliberately choose to change how you see yourself, what stress is, what failure is, even how you see the world around you, you come into consciousness and close the gap between power and fear as you wake up. Your awareness becomes an awakeness. Observing yourself, looking from the inside out rather than the outside in, changes everything.

The process of change requires you becoming
conscious of your unconscious self.

—Dr. Joe Dispenza

---

2. Work Diligently, Be Patient, and Take Baby Steps

*Any profound learning requires long stretches
of dedicated practice with no seeming progress.*

—Source unknown

If you are an athlete who has outbursts of anger in games and is trying to break the habit, how many moments of self-restraint will you have to demonstrate before you will have broken that habit and decide that you have adapted? When will the grains of sand become that new heap of desired change?

If you have been working on a new technique for your backhand swing in tennis, how many times will you have to be "unsuccessful" before you find success? When will you know your old technique has been replaced with the new one?

You must have a passionate dedication to the pursuit of short term goals. Change in sport most often happens in small bits: the aggregation of marginal gains, the Kaizen method of small steps. There will be a tipping point where the changing stops being a process and the change happens—when the grain of sand becomes that heap. The interesting thing is that most of us need less evidence to see decline and more to see improvement. A study out of the University of Chicago by Ed O'Brien and Nadav Klein discovered that there is a double standard in our perception of change: most of us hold the belief that change for the better is much more difficult than change for the worse. (Klein & O'Brien, 2017). That bias skews our ability to evaluate change. When we as athletes try to make a change, we tend to ignore signs of progress while interpreting signs of decline as real indications that there is no way to improve.

This creates a self-fulfilling prophecy. If you are working to improve as an athlete, and you don't see results as quickly as you would like, you may give up on something that could change your career. Do you recall a time when you gave up on something perhaps too quickly? If you decide that what you are doing is not working, soon it is not only your *perception* that what you are trying to change isn't working, it most certainly has become the *reality* because you have given up on it. Remember the Conscious Competence stages of learning? When we move to the second stage, where we know what we are supposed to do but cannot yet do it, we give up here more than at any other stage. Focusing on the benefits of learning rather than the process will keep you moving towards the change you desire.

I have talked about working on doing a handstand for a few years. It's something I have never been able to do. Some days I can hold it for a few seconds, other days not at all. I know what I need to do but cannot do it yet. I work diligently, not hard, and I use that word deliberately. Diligence implies working hard, but with a sense of doing things right, not hammering away with no method to your madness. Progress that I have made was not always noticeable. If I hadn't paid attention to the small improvements, I would have given up long ago. It certainly would have been easy to think I would never get it and give up, but I enjoy trying to figure out how to balance on my hands regardless of whether I actually do or not. The biggest lesson for me has been patience, not handstands; learning and practicing patience has helped me as an athlete and in all other aspects of my life.

> Do you recall a time when you gave up on something perhaps too quickly?

We confuse the truth that change requires effort with the myth that success is unlikely. If you are pushing that change, you most likely are right, that it is unlikely. Change can be hard, just like doing an Ironman can be hard, but the truth that it requires effort doesn't negate the fact that most of the people who commit to it, and are pulled toward it, will eventually succeed. Therein lies the place where the shift needs to happen—where you see the effort and commitment it requires to change as improving your chances of changing rather than making it unlikely. The effort of being drawn towards change rather than forcing it is much more likely to result in the change you desire.

We are what we repeatedly do. Excellence, then, is not an act, but a habit.

—Aristotle

---

3. Keep an Open Mind and Open Heart

Successful change results from a deliberate, intentional, powerful, and open mindset. It requires time in the uncomfortable, unfamiliar, uncertain, and unpredictable landscape of your body, mind, and heart.

The same way you can learn that new tennis backhand swing, you can learn to think in new ways. The circuitry of movement of the body will change with enough deliberate practice as will the circuitry of the movement of the mind. More often than not, what "feels" right to us is really just what is "familiar" to us. Moving out of familiarity and what feels right requires becoming comfortable in the unknown.

When you "know" something is wrong, you need to change that something. As long as that something you need to change "feels" right or familiar, until you delve into the unfamiliar, no change will be possible. Your logical "knowing" mind will override your "feeling" intuitive heart. We are all guilty of repeating the same pattern of movement, thoughts, and behavior, expecting a different outcome (change) and wondering why it doesn't happen. And we all know what that is the definition of, right? Yep. Insanity.

Your body has become the chemical result of your mind. When you look to "change your mind," your body will look to unseat those changes because it will be chemically uncomfortable. Even though you desire change, your desire for comfort will initially be stronger. It will be a process, and well worth it when you realize how the impossible becomes possible with the practice of an open mind and heart.

The Fifth Step towards consciousness is intentional generation of a positive state. The state of coherence—the highly efficient physiological state where the cardiovascular, nervous, hormonal, and immune systems are balanced, in sync, and work efficiently and harmoniously with energetic coordination—is tapped into through your heart and your emotions. It is a state of heart-brain synchronization where higher motor faculties and intuition equals a flow, liquid co-ordination, a way to exceed perceived limits in a magical and mystical state of deliberately altered consciousness.

As mentioned before, the electromagnetic field of the heart is the most powerful and extensive one in our bodies. When you learn to deliberately generate a coherent heart rhythm, a harmonious state of your mind and body, you change the landscape of your being and potential.

Emotions contribute to stress and can impair performance. Most athletes don't realize the emotional stresses that they habitually feel are the biggest inhibitors to performance. Feelings of pressure, doubt, anxiety, and failure can all become a habitual and familiar response to game day. Your emotional response to your event can do a lot of damage to your ability to perform up to your potential. Negative emotions trigger the brain, ANS, and hormonal systems to go into a fight-or-flight response. As discussed in the "Tiptoe Around Your Amygdala" section, having a high awareness of your emotions helps you change. Learning to generate positive emotions will be a process and take some time. If we had a delete key like our computers, it certainly would make it much easier to change a habit. Changes on a neural and hormonal level take time, awareness, and practice.

Emotions fuel a hormonal response in our bodies. Negative emotions fuel cortisol. When you have a bad shot in a game and you deal with it angrily, cortisol is pumped into your system. You may calm down your nervous system with the breath we have already discussed, but the cortisol sticks around for hours. DHEA is the "anti-aging" or "vitality" hormone. It is fueled by positive emotions. Just like cortisol, it will hang out in your body for hours. After that same "bad" shot, you can look at it with gratitude for the opportunity to learn something, pump DHEA into your system, and move forward in your game with potential for high performance rather than diminished.

To change the stress response, you simply use that same fuel that drives it: emotions. By consciously and deliberately building new emotional habits, you will change your perspective, change the outcome of your game, and even better, improve your health.

Change happens somewhere between 21 and 40 or even up to 254 days, with the average being 76, according to a study from University College London. (Lally, 2009). The important thing is that consistency and repetition are necessary to create new patterns and to learn to do things differently than you have in your past. It is easier to do something new than to stop a behavior without something to replace it. Whatever the new behavior you are looking to practice and to make a new habit will become your new "go to." One baby step at a time.

4. Practice "Undoing" and "Letting Go"...Lose your Mind

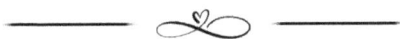

I wonder if there is a school of unlearning.

—Charlie Mackesy

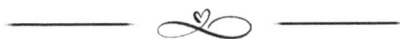

The first step towards consciousness is having awareness that you are unconscious, and the second step is having a beginner's mind. In understanding what isn't working for you, you make change possible by being open to new possibilities and letting go of preconceived notions or behaviors. You can only change what you notice. I have often called the process of change "the great undoing," like an unraveling of years of being bound up in what others have told us, what false beliefs we have of ourselves, of fear-based behaviors, and of living a life that we were told to live rather than consciously choosing how we decide to live.

You will have to get real with yourself and really know where you want to go. Be positive that you are going to make the changes necessary to head in that new direction. *I am keeping a calm, cool mindset during all golf matches regardless of how I play.* Having teammates, coaches, friends, and family commit to it with you certainly can help.

It can help to write down the outcome you desire. Measure everything you can and use the data to drive the change. *No outbursts of negativity, from throwing clubs to self-criticism.* You will experience resistance from yourself at first, and you must understand that it is fear of the unfamiliar driving that resistance. When you make your first bad drive after committing to this change, you won't know what to do or how to do it.

There will be a space, a gap between no longer displaying what you desire to change and not yet being able to implement what you are practicing changing. That space will be uncomfortable, unfamiliar, and will require conscious effort on your part in order to move through it. Living by choice rather than by chance requires practice.

Providing feedback and positive reinforcement, from yourself and from your support team, will help ensure success in your desired changes. Making the new choices pleasurable and the old ones costly and uncomfortable is important. Every time you make a bad shot and remain calm, celebrate! Have an "I didn't throw my golf club" dance. Throw your arms up in a victory V and cheer! Every time you make a bad shot and go back to old patterns, make yourself take the next three shots to your non-dominant side.

Dr. Joe Dispenza's book, *Breaking The Habit of Being Yourself— How to Lose Your Mind and Create a New One*, is a great read if you really want to look at how to make changes in your life. He combines the fields of quantum physics, neuroscience, brain chemistry, biology, and genetics to show you what is truly possible. He knows that change can come from pain and suffering or from joy and inspiration. In choosing to consciously change, we can expect to feel some discomfort, experience inconvenience and unpredictable routine, and will most definitely go through a period of not knowing.

Taking your inventory is the third step towards consciousness. After taking a look at the habits of who you "are" and beginning to create who you would like to "be" will require some introspection, not only in the sport you play, but in the life you are living. You may "lose your mind" when you hit a golf ball and it slices hard into the rough. On introspection, you understand that it isn't really losing your mind that is the problem, it is the habit you have of allowing anger to be the response to the mistake you made. Losing the mind that is holding on to that habit is the way to start down the road of making that change.

Envisioning a golf career plagued by broken clubs and being avoided by other players is often a more powerful motivation for choosing an emotion other than anger. Focusing on avoiding loss and raising the cost of bad behavior may be more motivating than attaining gain.

Set small, achievable, measurable goals. Abandoning beliefs and ideas that have been programmed into you for years will take time. If you don't let go of them, you most certainly will continue to be dragged down by them. Reward and acknowledge the small steps. The key to success is stringing together enough of the consciously chosen decisions.

5. Rewire Mental and Emotional Neural Circuitry

Habits are really just redundant sets of automatic, unconscious behaviors, thoughts, and emotions that you acquired through repetition. Recurring mental and emotional states become actual neural circuitry. You have done them over and over again so many times that your mind and body have wired the circuits into limited and finite patterns that become not only your habits, but have actually chiseled your identity. You are a set of hardwired, memorized behaviors, emotional reactions, and unconscious attitudes that you, or perhaps others, have programmed yourself to be. You can change by becoming aware of what you think about and becoming conscious of what patterns you have wired together.

To break free of those unconscious programs/patterns that have had a long held power over your actions and reactions, you will have to change your mind on the most basic level. You will have to see that your beliefs about cause and effect may either no longer be in accordance with what you want out of life or are standing in the way of the life you envision. If the wiring in your house is outdated and doesn't serve the new technology, you can only access that new technology by rewiring.

As we discussed earlier, simply visualizing or mentally rehearsing can start the installation of new neurological circuits and pathways in our brains. If you don't want to have emotional outbursts when you are performing badly, what thoughts and behaviors and feelings do you want to wire and fire together to demonstrate a more conscious response to that circumstance and environment?

Shutting down the wiring that no longer serves you and opening new wiring that serves the new you will make changes on behavioral and neurological levels. You have been unconsciously wiring your brain your whole life. When you step into awareness, you can chip away at what behaviors, thoughts, and feelings you want to disconnect from and start connecting new ones. Being able to observe yourself and intentionally affect change will move you towards the ideal version you have of yourself as an athlete and human being. Visualizing and mentally rehearsing who you want to be installs new wiring in your brain that creates the reality that it has already happened.

Deliberate practice with intentional excellence was Step Four in the path to consciousness. Not only deliberately and intentionally practicing your game but deliberately and intentionally practicing who you are while playing that game will lead you to a much more fulfilled and successful life.

6. Choose Your Emotions and Follow Them Into a Conscious Future

You can look at your emotions as an indicator of how your thoughts blend with what is really happening in your life. When you learn to consciously evoke positive emotions and know them "by heart" rather than unconsciously allowing old patterns that you know "by habit," you will have the power to live a much more coherent and powerful life.

In Step Five, I talked about the state of coherence and how consciously generating positive emotions through your heart is the way to achieve that. If you keep choosing the same thoughts and emotions, you are going to have the same behaviors, experiences, and outcomes. By becoming aware of what you think about (being the observer) and consciously choosing your emotions, you can decide what you are going to leave in your past and what you will bring into your future. It is not possible to keep your same personality *and* create a new reality. Change starts inside you, your heart and your mind, your chemistry and your electromagnetic fields.

Just like mentally rehearsing new thoughts to rewire your brain, you can rehearse new emotions to change your body and bring a future that you choose. Remember that what feels "right" to you is really just familiar. Throwing your golf club is just familiar for some reason you probably can't even figure out, but instead of choosing anger when you miss a shot, you can choose gratitude so your past behaviors disappear and new ones replace them in your future.

As discussed earlier, the magnetic field produced by the heart is more than 5,000 times greater in strength than the field generated by the brain and is detected several meters around the body. It is so powerful that the information it transmits can be received by the consciousness of others. It is scientifically evident that the heart's field is modulated by the emotional state of the individual. (McCraty, 2015). Learning to reprogram your heart with conscious and intentional emotions is most certainly a power with which to be reckoned. There is often a gap or a disagreement between what the brain and the heart intend.

When that gap is big, you are operating unconsciously. Intention was a tool I talked about earlier. If you *intend* to make changes but the gap between the brain and heart stays wide, the likelihood of that change happening diminishes. Remember that intentions have to feel good, and if they don't, they are less likely to happen. There is too big of a gap between the heart and brain. If you *know* you should change, but don't, the culprit may also be that gap. When you find the right intention point, when the meeting ground of the mind and heart are synchronized, you are able to change your experiences in the future and rewire your emotional memory.

There is technology I use for myself and my athletes to help them see the power of choosing their emotions to develop coherence. The Inner Balance™ and em®Wave technologies of HeartMath® analyze and display your heart rhythm, measured by HRV, which indicates how emotional states are affecting your nervous system. High performance is about turning stress into coherence. Inner Balance is a tool you can use on your phone or tablet that allows you to practice stress intervention techniques and objective biometric feedback that quantifiably and dramatically boosts your health and your performance.

Anna Hemmings, a former Olympian and World Champion flat-water kayaker for the UK, taught a HeartMath® Certification for Sports Professionals that I attended in 2015 that showed how the tools of HeartMath® could be used to enhance performance. Not only could you learn to control your physiology and psychology, you could see in real time how you operated when competing to get a better under-standing of yourself as an athlete. She used me to demonstrate how the technology could teach coaches and athletes about their emotional states while performing.

First, she asked the group to write a brief story of three com-petitions we had been in. Not knowing what any of us wrote, she asked me to demonstrate the em®WavePro technology that is used on a desktop. I was to close my eyes, feel myself going through each race, and if she asked me at any time what was happening, to give her one descriptive word. The first race I visualized was Ironman New Zealand. I went through the race in a condensed version and as I was close to the finish line in my mind, she said, "What is happening?" and I said, "I'm finishing." She told me to go to my next event, which was an Olympic distance triathlon in which I had won the masters women's age group. Again, I went through my race and as I approached the finish line, she asked what was happening. I was very interested in how she seemed to know when I was close to finishing—what was this technology showing her? The third event was a Sprint distance triathlon that I won overall women's. I went through the race in my mind and again, Anna asked what was happening as I was finishing.

She told me that I was an athlete that enjoyed the journey, not the outcome, which is very true. But how did she know that from the data? My coherence varied as I went through each race, and shifted in some way that showed her when I crossed the finish line in my mind. This technology gave insight to things I wanted to know about my own athletes. Understanding coherence was a way to understand how to enhance performance on a whole other level.

I have used Inner Balance™ on many of my clients, from stroke patients to Ironman athletes. Seeing real time how we have control over our physiology is quite empowering. Using it personally helped me see how my mantra of keeping my head in my own boat really did enhance my performance. Indoor computrainer classes with a large group of cyclists was a place where you could see data from pace to power on a big screen at the front of the class. Riding with the Inner Balance™ technology, I could immediately see when I looked at what was going on around me instead of what was going on inside me, my power, pace, and coherence would immediately drop.

Understanding that you have choice when it comes to emotion when competing may not be something you have considered or even believe. Seeing the reprogramming with the aid of technology like this will most certainly raise your awareness. It can help encourage you to reconsider and start shifting your beliefs.

TOOL #6:
DE-STRESS AND RE-COVER

———— ⚬—∞ ————

*It is not stress that kills us, but our reaction to
it. Adopting the right attitude can convert a
negative stress into a positive one. Man should
not try to avoid stress any more than he would
shun food, love, or exercise.*

—Hans Selye

———— ⚬—∞ ————

Stress + Avoidance/Resistance = More Stress
Stress + Adaptation/Reflection = Progress

Stress is more than a momentary reaction for many of us. It's a habit. The effects of it don't grow overnight. They build over a lifetime, over a career.

Releasing stress requires reversing ingrained habits, and that takes time and awareness. Time and awareness softens the resistance we build to challenging realities, a resistance that is deeply encoded in our physical, mental, and emotional attachments and perceptions. Time and awareness rewires the brain pathways that would normally go into the reactive stress response, facilitates growth of new attitudes, and creates new habits that feel good to ensure lasting change.

With this ever-increasing pace of life, we try harder and harder to keep up with the chaos and busyness of the world around us. I call this effort: *exstress*. It defines the stress overload produced by the overwhelming amount of responsibilities many of us take on and the resulting feeling of loss of control over our life and personal situations. Stress is most often a fear response, not a rational reply that triggers negative thoughts and emotions. When we believe it is happening *to* us, we become victims of it. When we understand how it is happening *in* us, we can reduce the physiological and psychological effects. What we *are* in control of is this: deliberately preparing for what *can* happen and then responding with conscious intent to what *does* happen. Why is recognizing and dealing with stress so important to us as athletes?

Developing the ability to manage stress, along with using techniques to consciously turn the stress response down, helps our bodies move into recovery mode. It may be the missing piece in most of our lives that can help elevate energy levels, increase recovery ability, and enhance performance. If your rate of recovery improves as you start to pay more attention to your body, higher training volumes and intensities will be possible without the detriment of overtraining.

Hans Selye was a pioneer in the field of stress. As a medical student, he observed identical signs and symptoms in patients that were suffering from different diseases. He said they just "looked sick." As a result of those and many other observations, he coined the word "stress" and defined it as "a non-specific response of the body to a demand." (Selye, 1936). Interestingly enough, he later expressed his

General Adaptation Syndrome

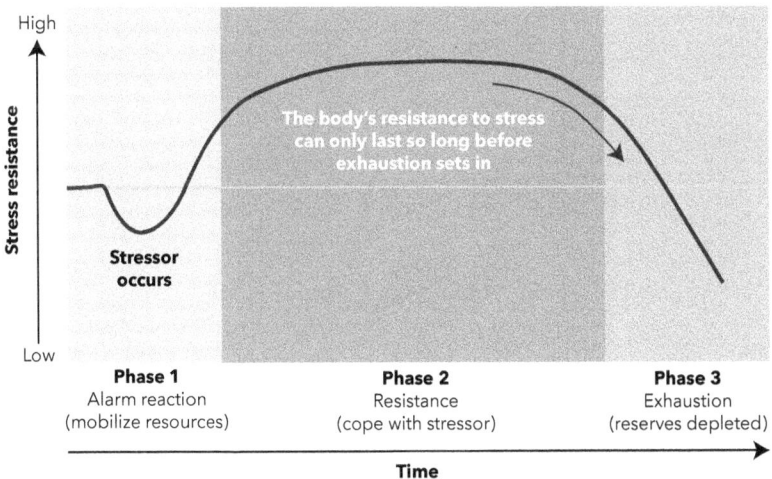

High

Stress resistance

The body's resistance to stress can only last so long before exhaustion sets in

Stressor occurs

Low

Phase 1	**Phase 2**	**Phase 3**
Alarm reaction	Resistance	Exhaustion
(mobilize resources)	(cope with stressor)	(reserves depleted)

Time

lack of knowledge of the English language and in retrospect, said he would have used the word "strain" instead.

He later discovered and described the General Adaptation Syndrome, a response of the body to demands placed upon it. The syndrome details how stress induces hormonal autonomic responses and, over time, these hormonal changes can lead to health issues including ulcers, high blood pressure, arteriosclerosis, arthritis, kidney disease, and allergic reactions. His seminal work, *A Syndrome Produced by Diverse Nocuous Agents,* was published in 1936 in *Nature.* (Selye, 1936).

Stress is a natural condition in which the human system responds to changes in its normal, balanced state. A stressor is anything that is perceived as challenging, threatening, or demanding, and adaptation is the change that takes place as a result of the response to a stressor. Adaptation is a physiological principle that is one of the truths of exercise science.

You simply cannot be an athlete without stress. Exercise is a physiological stressor, regardless of the load. Our bodies need to be challenged in order to get stronger, fitter, faster, and leaner. When you adequately and appropriately increase load on the bodily systems that respond to training, they adapt. Too little stress and there is no adaptation; we may even become fragile. Too much stress and we risk our body breaking down; we become injured and fatigued. The trick is to find the adequate amount of stress paired with the appropriate amount of recovery.

Let's take a look at what knocks us out of that sweet spot.

Overloading

There are three levels of overtraining or overloading.

1. Functional overreaching that is necessary to make improvements and must be paired with sufficient recovery.

2. Non-functional overreaching that will require excess recovery time to get the full benefit. The body will require extra time to repair itself from the excess stress.
3. Overtraining syndrome is marked by significant detriment to health and performance. Both functional and nonfunctional over-reaching can lead to overtraining if insufficient rest is paired with it. Symptoms like increased injury, abnormal hormone levels, depression, and mental stress are inevitable and in some athletes are ignored, perhaps because their training is more of a coping strategy or escape rather than a way to enhance performance.

If you are using sport as a Band-Aid to hide false, fear-based beliefs about yourself, any setback in training will only expose the wound under that Band-Aid. Increasing your awareness of your body, your training behaviors, and your ability to tolerate load will help you stay functional in your training practices. Overload also happens when you believe the "more is better" myth. Thinking that what you do in your training is never enough will inevitably lead to doing more. Always doing more will inevitably lead to overtraining.

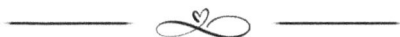

It takes courage to say yes to rest and play in a culture where exhaustion is seen as a status symbol.

—Brené Brown

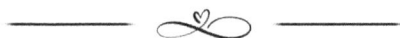

Selye identified two kinds of stress. *Eustress* is positive; it is man-ageable stress that can lead to growth and enhanced competence. It is both challenging and uncomfortable but leads to health and adap-tation. *Distress* is negative in that it goes beyond discomfort and into pain. When uncontrolled, prolonged, and overwhelming, it can be destructive. The line between the two can be very subjective. It has more to do with how you perceive and react to your situation than what the situation really is. The same experience for one person can be a healthy challenge while being overly stressful for another. (Selye, 1936).

Our bodies will tell us through fatigue, diminished performance, illness, and injury when they are distressed. We tend to ignore those messages when we think that we should be able to handle more stress. We turn eustress into distress by going beyond the limits of our bodies without giving enough recovery, when we go beyond overreaching to overtraining. We resist the notion that perhaps less is better at some points in our training rather than more. How do you know when stress is enough or too much? You must pay close attention to your body to listen when it tells you that you are at the edge of tolerance and to not go beyond that point.

Selye called this unconscious pattern "maladaptive coping," where strategies to deal with stress further exacerbate the problem rather than solve it. (Selye, 1936). Going beyond the edges of tolerance will inevitably sideline you with injury and illness. When you have been diagnosed with bilateral tibial stress fractures after running through pain while training for the marathon you "have" to run, I would suggest you need to revisit your coping techniques. A better solution is "adaptive coping," which contributes to resolution of the stress response. You may not enjoy "water running" or canceling your marathon, but running on broken shins only pushes you into more distress, deeper into maladaptive coping, and into a preservation response where your body will eventually "win" with more injury or illness. Believe me, I learned that with some hard lessons.

One of my favorite definitions of stress is "our resistance to our own lives." We all know people who are always stressed, overwhelmed, and fight the life they are living day in and day out. Then, we know those who look at the glass as half full, see the silver lining, and live each day of their lives as it unfolds, with gratitude. Consider which of those people you are. The JAMA Intern Med Journal in 2013 stated that "60–80% of primary care doctor visits are related to stress, yet only 3% of patients receive stress management help." (Nerurkar, 2013). Everything from depression to strokes, headaches to panic disorders, obesity to chronic fatigue can be the result of not dealing with the stress in our lives in an adaptive coping way. Finding tools to help "ease" your way through, rather than resist, the stresses of your life, will ensure less "dis-ease."

The greatest weapon against stress is our ability to choose one thought over another.

—William James

The third kind of stress can be considered "artificial" or "perceived" stress: that resistance you have to what is going on in your life. Your body cannot distinguish stress that is in your mind from actual stress. Stress happens *in* us, far more than *to* us. Athletes who understand that their thoughts about an error in their game are actually more of a problem than the error itself can move forward and fix the error more readily. Learning how to evaluate performance in a productive way, plan for disruptions, and shift into positive change can eliminate artificial stress rather than add to it.

> Stress happens *in* us far more than *to* us.

The more conscious you are about your passion for your sport and your underlying motivations, the more you will reduce artificial stress. Understanding that who you are is not defined by whether you win or lose can significantly reduce perceived stress. If you are unconsciously using sport as a way to cope, your resistance to losing can be a devastating and stressful situation. And those wins? They can be just as stressful when you discover they are a short term high, not a long term fix.

What follows is a list of strategies to reduce stress and enhance recovery. Some have been previously stated in the book, and I feel are very much worth repeating. As your awareness increases as a conscious athlete, you may find that intentional rest aids your performance more than you previously believed.

How to Deal with and Reduce Stress

1. Listen to your body; know *your* edge
2. Take your HRV daily
3. Reduce inflammation
4. Evoke positive emotions in negative situations
5. Be mindful; meditate
6. Open the gate of your RAS; be the creator of your life
7. Build resistance
8. Breathe
9. Deliberately rest and recover
10. Take rest seriously
11. Save your mental energy

1. Listen to your body; know your edge

Our bodies work miracles every day. Our hearts beat 100,000 times, pumping 2,000 gallons of blood a day. (Texas Heart Institute). About 330 billion cells are replaced daily. (Scientific American, 2021). A new skeleton is made every 5–10 years (Cleveland Clinic, 2022) along with a new layer of skin every 40–56 days. (Koster, 2009). We take about 22,000 breaths a day. (Breathing, 2014).

And that is what it does without us even having to think about it or work at it. All the while, it fixes every cut, wound, broken bone, and fights off illnesses without you even knowing. Even when you give more to it than it can handle, it is still there for you, working to keep you alive, breathing, and as healthy as it can.

Your body does its very best and it listens to you. Oftentimes, as athletes, we ask it to do more than it possibly can. Our bodies will respond and adapt given the opportunity after being asked, but only if we don't push them to the point of distress.

The wonderful thing about our body is that often, it will give us early warnings of impending illness and injury. It won't lie, and it won't exaggerate. It will be clear and specific. It is the quiet voice with the most important message. The whispers of being out of balance, over-trained, under-recovered, if listened to, will resolve. When not listened to, the whispers will become loud voices, even yelling to get our attention to stop, rest, and recover. Believe me, I know from experience. I am sure that some of you reading this book have suffered your own consequences of ignoring what your body tried to tell you. A mind that doesn't listen to the body is more like a bully than a training partner.

Please consider giving the same attention you give to the data of your training to the data of your recovery. Technology now allows us to measure improvements in performance, and we pour over that data, relentlessly trying to make further improvements. Our heart rates, speed, power, strength, agility, and technique are all diligently recorded and used to further push our limits. We can also use technology to recover more fully and keep our bodies in a state of health rather than on the edge of injury or disease.

There is a fine line sometimes between pushing and finding your edge or going over that edge. Knowing your body and where that line is keeps you in the competition rather than taking you out. Using heart rate training zones can be a great metric to direct your training. Using heart rate as a guide, rather than the pace or speed you think you should be going, is a way for your physiology to work in your favor as opposed to your ego working against you. Sometimes you must go faster to get faster, and other times it is better to go slower to get faster.

Developing a conscious awareness of your body and its ability to recover and handle load is part of taking your performance to new levels. Learning to listen for feedback and honoring the cues it gives you is respecting its intelligence. Staying unconscious and denying, overriding, or suppressing symptoms will only cause your body to break down even further and make performing to your ability impossible. Once something in your body "breaks," it is a long and sometimes impossible process to get it back to where it was. Subtle joint pain that is ignored may become a need for surgery. Cold symptoms that are ignored can lower your ability to fight other infections. When your ego and perhaps your addiction to your sport drive the vehicle of your body, there is most certainly going to be a crash.

Where is the line for you between challenge and overtraining? If you have a strong understanding of the difference between functional overreaching and overtraining, you most likely don't spend too much time trying to put all the broken pieces of yourself back together to be able to compete at your potential. When you understand what it takes for your body to adapt to the load you put on it rather than exhaust it continually because you ignore or don't know your edge, you have the ability to perform optimally. Chronic levels of stress and overtraining will not only diminish your performance, they will diminish your health.

> Where is the line for you between challenge and overtraining?

Pushing your edge can have big payoffs in the short term, but long term it will come with a high cost and potentially create debt that can bankrupt your athletic career.

That edge will be different for you and for everyone else. That edge may move back and forth on a day-to-day basis, in different stages of your training, and ages of your life. Overtraining may be more of a sliding scale than a line and does not follow any clear-cut rules. If you handled over-distance and interval training for your last marathon five years ago, it doesn't necessarily mean that is the right plan to follow now. In those five years, you may have been completely sedentary, had a couple of children (and therefore most likely less sleep), or taken up tennis because you lost your enthusiasm for running.

The earlier you start to create balance in your stress response, the higher the likelihood that injury and illness will not be a factor in your ability to train and perform. Finding that balance and tapping into your conscious awareness may allow you to realize that all the attention you have been giving to your physical body and your outside achievements helped to create that immense load of stress on your body and your life. To achieve your greatest potential, your efforts to reduce that load may lead you inward and help you understand there is more to you on the inside than the outside.

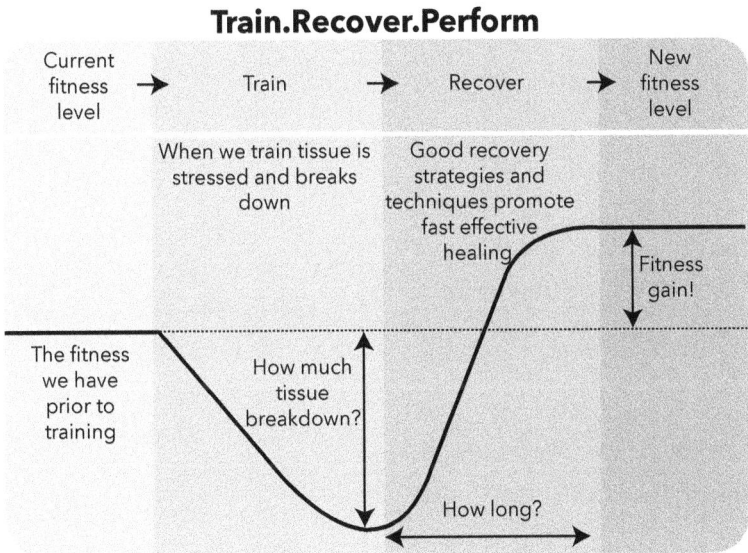

Train.Recover.Perform

Current fitness level	→	Train	→	Recover	→	New fitness level

When we train tissue is stressed and breaks down

Good recovery strategies and techniques promote fast effective healing

Fitness gain!

The fitness we have prior to training

How much tissue breakdown?

How long?

2. Take your HRV daily

Choosing to practice rising above the chaos and stress in your life will help you maintain your resilience, energetic balance, and health. Learning to tap into the heart's natural guidance and intuitive direction results in smarter choices and better outcomes in your performance and life.

We know that having a high heart rate variability (HRV) is important with regards to coping with stress as an athlete. Not just learning to only load your body to manageable levels but also keeping a positive emotion and attitude when dealing with the stresses of your sport and training, are tools you can use to keep yourself in adaptation rather than exhaustion.

Seeing stress as a challenge rather than a threat can be a game changer.

HRV provides the brain with information about your external environment and how it is being perceived. This basically allows the brain to keep you alive. If you are about to walk off a cliff and you are not processing the danger, you will keep walking and fall to your death. If you ignore that you are fatigued, unable to perform at optimal levels, and injured more often than not, you just may be ignoring the cliff of overtraining and not understand how you fell off. HRV is a non-invasive measure of your autonomic nervous system and provides insight as to how your brain is regulating your body based on the pattern your heart is beating in. It is a powerful predictor of performance along with health and wellness. Basically, a higher HRV shows the body has a strong ability to tolerate stress or is strongly recovering from accumulated stress. Your brain perceives the pattern of your heart and responds accordingly.

> As you increase your training load, you decrease your ability to train harder. You must recover from your increased load, not train harder in order to improve your performance. This is a very important concept to wrap your mind around.

You can use HRV on a daily basis to track your response to the stresses of training and learn to not only improve your performance, but also to manage and predict it. Just as you have a threshold with regards to heart rate, strength, and power, you also have a training threshold of how much load you can handle at any given point in your training.

As you increase your training load, you decrease your ability to train harder. You must recover from your increased load, not train harder in order to improve your performance. This is a very important concept to wrap your mind around. Training too much above your threshold leads you into *preservation response* rather than *training response*. In that preservation response, there is not enough recovery and too much stress, and the body will eventually shut down. When there is a balance between stress and recovery, the body and its performance will improve.

Your body is an adaptive organism. To deal with a chronic imbalance of stress and recovery from that stress, in order to protect itself from harm, it will most definitely diminish your ability to perform. Just as too little stress or training will not improve performance, too much will do the same.

3. Reduce inflammation

Chronic inflammation in our bodies relates to disease. Signs of chronic inflammation according to the latest findings include depression/anxiety/brain fog, stomach pain, and being tired even when you get enough sleep.

When you are in your SNS, there is an inflammatory response from the adrenaline release that is normal and important, but when we get locked into a chronic inflammatory state, we move from health to disease. The human body is not designed to have adrenaline and cortisol flowing through it for extended periods of time. The PNS stimulates our vagus nerve and suppresses the inflammatory response when it releases acetylcholine. This is when adaptation takes place. If you don't spend time there, you go into exhaustion.

Studies have shown that HRV is inversely related to inflammatory markers. HRV provides a gauge of your body's ability to regulate inflammation effectively that results from the stresses of our lives including poor sleep, poor nutrition, and over training. Tracking your HRV gives you an inside look at your overall inflammation and resulting health and wellness or disease and illness.

Chronic inflammation is the hallmark of metabolic syndromes like type 2 diabetes, hypertension, and cardiovascular disease. Chronic inflammation also promotes fat storage. If your calorie intake is too low and your stress is too high, you will gain fat, because chronic inflammation causes fat storage instead of fat loss. When inflammation is high and HRV is low because of the stresses of overtraining, poor nutrition, lack of sleep, or an over-demanding lifestyle, you will not be able to remain healthy or perform optimally. Chronic inflammation creates the perfect place for illness, injury, disease, and the inability to perform to your potential.

When you practice better recovery from your training, eat well, sleep deeply, and live authentically, you will reduce the inflammatory response and increase your HRV.

4. Evoke positive emotions in perceived negative situations

Remember the formula, Performance = Potential – Interference? There is no way around that math.

The quality of emotions that we create within our heart determines the signal that we send to the brain, which in turn releases chemicals into our bodies. The conversation between our heart and brain can be healing or toxic, healthy or stressful. Emotions will always win over logic. When negative emotions interfere with your potential, performance is inevitably affected. Managing emotions is something you can practice and learn to do to improve your performance.

If you recall the Fifth Step to consciousness, intentionally generating a positive state ensures that your neuro-emotional brain enhances your neuro-logical brain. Generating a positive state not only reduces interference, but with practice, reduces the amount of stress you feel when your game or race doesn't go as planned.

5. Be mindful and meditate

I have already spoken about the tool of meditation and its benefits. Mindful meditation creates changes in the structure of the brain resulting in enhanced self-regulation, attention control, emotional regulation, and self awareness. (Tang, 2020). Those are valuable skills for athletes developing their introspective process.

Learning to quiet your mind is a practice in and of itself. Becoming mindful of what passes through your mind and heart—consciousness—is another practice. It is a way to notice what you are thinking or feeling and how that might add to that third type of stress, your perception of your reality. Being aware of what is going on in your mind without getting carried away by it or acting on it is important for athletes who want to perform their best. Responding consciously rather than reacting blindly and unconsciously can be a game changer.

That voice inside our head tells us a story based on our past and can be a huge factor in the amount of stress we experience. Rarely do our thoughts and feelings have anything to do with what is actually going on, but rather with what we focus on and *think* is going on. Negative thoughts create stress in our bodies. Our bodies cannot distinguish between our perceptions and reality and will respond according to what we think is real.

6. Open the gate of your RAS; be the creator of your life

You are always creating your future. You bring it forth through your thoughts, actions, feelings, beliefs, values, goals, and dreams. You do this regardless of the level of your conscious awareness. Your present moment awareness coupled with the future that you create is a deeper reflection of your subconscious programming. All of your future goals and dreams are not only a reflection of your subconscious thinking, they are also mediated by your Reticular Activating System (RAS). The RAS is the part of your brain that serves as a filter between your conscious mind and your subconscious mind. The RAS, which is located in the core of your brain stem, takes instructions from your conscious mind and passes them on to your subconscious mind. (Hallbom, 2012).

Have you ever been in the situation where something new comes into your life, maybe a new bike, and suddenly, that same make and model of bike is everywhere you look, and you never even noticed it before? Or maybe, you believe your teammates don't appreciate you enough, and all you hear is their criticism? These things happen because of an area in our brain called the Reticular Activating System or RAS which is an important enabling factor for our state of consciousness, behavior, arousal, and motivation. (Sang Seok Yeo, 2013). It filters out what it deems to be unnecessary, so important and familiar stuff gets through. So if you decide to focus on a goal, or decide to see the positive in things, your RAS automatically creates that filter for you. It helps you see what you want to see. It's like a gatekeeper and will often prevent contradictory information from what you already possess from being processed. Meditation is a way to open your mind and awareness and therefore that gate, for new possibilities to be considered.

The RAS also seeks out information that validates your beliefs. It filters the world through the parameters you give it and your beliefs shape. If you believe your teammates don't appreciate you, your RAS does its best to help you see exactly that.

The good news is you can train your RAS. If you think back to the chapters about intention, it makes even more sense that when you consciously set an intention, when you see your goals successfully, when you step into the role of director of the movie of your life, you are telling your RAS you expect it to happen. Just like the projector in Chapter 2, when you change the film, your brain—and this time, your RAS—you shape your reality consciously.

Learning to initially notice and then let go of that negative voice, while deliberately directing your mind and heart to see the bigger picture, is an important step in becoming more consciously in control of your life. It will not only help reduce the stress response and resulting inflammation, but help you become the creator of your reality rather than the victim of it.

Living as a victim creates a paradigm called the dreaded drama triangle (DDT), where the only two ways to see people or events in your life, as persecutor/persecution or rescuer/rescuing. Victims relinquish responsibility for their lives; life happens *to* them. Living as a creator through the empowerment dynamic (TED*), you see through the lens of challengers/challenges and coaches/empowerers. (David Emerald, 2016). You see possibility and your own potential and take charge of your life.

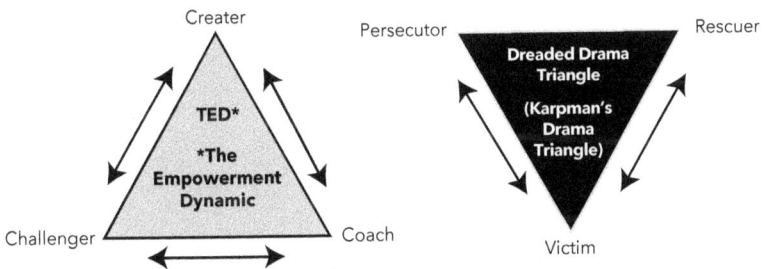

What happens in your life is not always your choice, but how you react to it is. You can choose to respond with stress or choose to be grateful for the lesson that situation teaches you. When you can learn to find the positive in any situation, to be fully present and open to what is happening and evoke gratitude, you are on your way to discovering what is possible. Sometimes what is required is a little patience, along with revisiting the negative you think is happening. What is happening to you may be happening *for* you.

I certainly have had my share of opportunities to learn those lessons and had that roommate-in-my-head impacting my stress levels. In 2005, five years after Ironman New Zealand, I went to race at Ironman Canada thinking I was ready and able to place high enough in my age group to qualify for the World Championships in Kona, Hawaii. The day handed me a whole other experience that challenged that roommate-in-my-head and my relationship with her. I can look back now and see that going into that day, there was so much stress on so many levels that I hadn't dealt with—*extress*. The stress of demanding my body to perform at elite levels to the stresses of being a single mom running a small business, combined with not giving myself even remotely enough recovery, finally caught up with me.

I wrestled the whole day with a sense that something was wrong. My head was not in the game, my body felt tired and sluggish, and my times for the swim and bike certainly confirmed for me that there was no chance I was going to Kona. By the time I got off the bike, I should have been halfway through the marathon. The stress I felt in so many ways seems ridiculous now that I have learned the lessons from that race. That roommate-in-my-head kept telling me to push through, that I had to prove myself to everyone, and what would they think if I didn't finish the race? They would think I was a loser, not good enough, someone who gave up. There was no option 14 miles into the 26.2 mile run other than to put an end to the race. After a long day of struggle that resulted in fluids coming out of both ends of my body, I finally had to listen to a voice of reason instead of that roommate. If I had not, I would have most certainly ended up in the medical tent.

And do you know what happened?

Failure turned into growth. What my mental roommate told me was failure became the biggest opportunity for growth. No longer did

I have to prove myself worthy to anyone, especially myself. I was enough regardless, because of knowing when to stop that day. I got to choose gratitude for the lesson and see that what was really happening was not in my head or on that race course, but in my heart and soul and in my openness to growth.

7. Build your resilience

Dealing with the physical stress we put on our bodies and adapting to it are two things we can learn to do better. Perhaps more importantly is dealing with the other stresses of life including emotional, financial, relational, professional, or environmental issues. The less resistance you put up to the reality of your life, the more you realize you are in control of your reaction to the world. The more opportunities you see in any situation, the less "stressed" you will be. Adaptability is the way to reduce resistance and deal with the perceived problems and difficulties. If you show up to race day and are presented with equipment malfunction, extreme weather conditions, or some opponent who "rattles your cage," that race might be over before it has even begun because of your inability to adapt.

Change and loss are unavoidable. In the adaptability and ease in which we experience change lies our happiness and freedom.

—Buddha

Resilience has begun to replace the term mental toughness. Toughness implies never showing vulnerability or weakness, while resiliency is regarded as the ability to persevere and to overcome perceived adversity and setbacks; the ability to overcome failures and barriers to achieve goals. Like a rubber ball, it implies a sort of "bounce back" ability. Attempting to bounce back will result in burnout if you do not take time to rest and recover. Resilience is built on growing in a rhythm of stress and recovery. It is a norm among successful athletes and can be practiced.

Resilience grows when you become intentional about bringing your best to the difficult situations in life. Stress is a signal to call on your resourcefulness, your intelligence, your courage. If you habitually see challenging situations as something being wrong rather than opportunity for growth, stress will win. If you see struggle and productive failure as the driving force of your work rather than the consequences of it, you are pushing at the point of resistance for growth rather than backing away from it. Difficulties don't paralyze you; instead, you learn from them.

Resilience results from the belief that you can be a positive force in your life and in the lives of others. It is a norm among successful people. It is not something you necessarily have; it includes thoughts, actions, and behaviors based on the belief that anyone can learn. Athletes who are resilient are most likely aligned with their goals and themselves. They have figured out how to deal with difficulty and distress. They are not pushing harder than their bodies can handle without allowing enough recovery.

We all know those athletes who have been in the game for decades with a race calendar that would seem impossible to most of us. Despite the apparently grueling schedule, they have the appearance of very low stress levels. Perhaps it is genetics, or their load of manageable stress is higher than most, or they have practiced seeing crisis as an opportunity and have learned to accept or deal with the things they cannot change. Perhaps they take three months off a year to not train, or they spend more time listening to their bodies than they do forcing them to perform.

Resilience and grit are qualities that enhance performance, no matter how successful or unsuccessful the performance might be. The thing about building resiliency is that athletes must face and learn to deal with adversity in order to conquer it in future events. If you strike out in the third inning of a baseball game and step up to the plate in the fourth inning carrying that strike-out with you, chances are you will repeat that error. It takes practice to stay in the present moment rather than stuck in a past failure. Performance errors can deteriorate confidence and cause athletes to lose control of their thoughts and emotions. The ability to let go of failure or to see it in a new light is key to future success.

Learning how to clear your mind will require developing new skills to bring you into the present. Perhaps stepping away from the plate and adjusting your gloves or helmet will remind you to be present for the pitch coming at you next rather than being stuck in your strike out of the last inning. Learning to let go of mistakes and managing your thoughts and emotions under pressure will build the resiliency to perform your best by learning to conquer any adversity or stressful situation. You build your emotional vitality and your ability to manage stress when you learn to choose the experience of positive thoughts and emotions.

Here is something to help you gauge your level of resilience in a given moment.

Your emotions are an indicator of how your thoughts blend with what is really happening in your life. Resisting what is happening creates unnecessary stress. Learning to evoke positive emotions and to empty your mind allows you to see things as they are rather than what you perceive them to be.

It's a very hot day. You are on the court playing tennis against a very formidable opponent, down to the last set for the win of the match. You are feeling overwhelmed, angry, ready to be done, and thinking about all the mistakes you made in the past five sets. Chances are, your emotions have put you into a reactive state; the serve about to come at you is likely to be the one that wins for your opponent when you don't return it.

You can turn that emotional state around: be grateful for the lessons you learned in every point you lost, understand that the heat is something everyone had to deal with that day, be present in that serve regardless of what the score is, do your best, and accept the outcome. It makes for a lot less stress than the previous scenario, and helps build that resiliency as you move forward in your athletic career.

The capacity to experience positive emotions may be a fundamental human strength central to the study of human flourishing.

—Barbara Fredrickson

Resilience can be built when you have support and a positive outlook. You can also cultivate it when you are open to learning new things, even as you make errors in learning, as long as you practice your beginner's mind. Knowing you are not perfect helps. Keeping your "head in your own boat" or "staying in your own lane" while taking control of and responsibility for your situation allows you to stay focused on what you want. Athletes who see their hard work as a choice rather than a sacrifice also generally see a setback in their performance as an opportunity for growth. Acting instead of reacting goes a long way, too. Resiliency is most certainly not going to be built if you allow your thoughts and subsequent reactions to go down the rabbit hole of negativity.

If you have been preparing for a big competition and your performance does not go as well as planned, you can be frustrated, angry, and upset while accepting responsibility. If you take the time to understand how and why you didn't perform as expected and understand how to plan to correct it in future events, then you can execute that plan the next time you perform. It can even be done as you're performing, if something as simple as the third hole of your golf game goes awry, and you don't want to carry that into the next 15 holes. Learning to see a "bad" event as temporary goes a long way to viewing whatever happens next in an optimistic light.

Resilient athletes see everything as an opportunity for self-discovery. Instead of reacting with the fight-or-flight response and allowing their amygdala to drive their behavior, they choose caution and curiosity, and are aware of choices they have to act. They are challenged by tough circumstances, not victimized by them. They know not to approach problems with the same thinking that created them and to accept that change is a mandatory part of life.

Just like our bodies have an immune system, our brains have a *psycho-immune* system. Just as you can build immunity in your body, you can also build immunity in your brain. What you eat, your attitude, a healthy lifestyle, reduced stress, sleep, sleep, and more sleep all build immunity in the body and brain.

Resilient athletes often take care of themselves with healthy nutrition, adequate water intake, and especially plenty of quality sleep. They step forward and take action to deal with problems and step back to rest and recharge. They have a good support system, know it takes small steps towards big goals, and take decisive actions when they need to. They have the ability to manage emotions, especially in stressful situations. Communication and problem-solving are skills they work on, and they have a positive view of themselves and their strengths.

They are also less reactive to their reality. They know that something that triggers a negative reaction is really their own fault. They are creators, not victims. If your habit is to view challenging situations as though something is wrong, you will be highly reactive. Learning to create a gap between stimulus and response, to have time to process and deliberately act, results in power and reduces stress.

> Increase the space between
>
> stimulus   and   response.
>
> Act. Don't react.

In that space between stimulus and response, mindfulness and awareness are crucial. When you are able to observe yourself, notice your thoughts, feelings, and behaviors, you can respond deliberately instead of unconsciously. It will be an uncomfortable place at first, that space. Those demons that have been chasing you, those maladaptive coping skills you unconsciously use, will cbe there to meet you. It will demand more from you than your physical training ever could. When you invite yourself into that space and navigate a new course of action, you will have found a conscious shift in the way you perform in your sport and live your life.

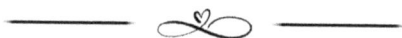

———— ♥ ————

Between stimulus and response there is a space.
In that space is our power to choose our response.
In our response lies our growth and our freedom.

—Viktor Frankl

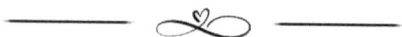

———— ♥ ————

Passion for your sport without grit or resilience will not bring you the success you desire. There will be ebbs and flows over your life as an athlete, and if you cannot remain committed to your goals no matter what, if you cannot see the long-term vision and passion, you most certainly will lose that passion with no foundation of stamina to stand on. When you learn to be grateful for the challenges you have, you increase your resilience, open up to growth, and tap into a mindset that helps you find creative solutions to problems you encounter. With the lens of gratitude, difficulties in life become opportunities to grow and move towards your goals with resilience.

8. Breathe and Practice Yoga

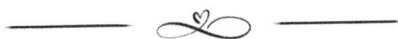

Stress is basically a disconnection from the earth,
a forgetting of the breath. Stress is an ignorant state.
It believes everything is an emergency.

—Natalie Goldberg

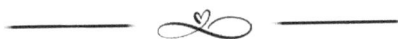

I have said a lot already about breathing. I want to remind you again about its value in reducing our stress, because it is worth repeating. Emotional stress can cause all kinds of problems: moodiness, anxiety, depression, irritability, and feelings of pressure, along with physical symptoms like headaches, stomach problems, and even chest pain. It can decrease our ability to empathize, deplete our energy levels, and often causes a disconnect and isolation from the things and people we love. Some of these symptoms are clearly consistent with overtraining. If your sport is causing you stress, you might want to look at your emotional patterns of response.

That stress you feel, perhaps from the pressure to perform at a level you are not ready for, will cause an erratic heart rate which sets off a decrease in your psychophysiological coherence level. Understanding that your heart responds to your breathing means you can change the landscape of the stress you perceive with deliberate, conscious, slow breaths. Breathing slowly and mindfully triggers the hypothalamus to stimulate the pituitary gland to send out stress reducing hormones and trigger a relaxation response in the body.

There are many breathing methods to induce change in the body. Yoga has a library of methods called *pranayama—prana*, breath; *yama*, control—as a way to attain higher awareness. Breath is about more than inhaling and exhaling; it is also about holding the breath, or breath retention (as discussed earlier in practicing CO_2 tolerance). One to start with that is quite simple is the 4-7-8 technique.

- Inhale for 4 counts through your nose, with your tongue on the back of your teeth.
- Hold for 7 counts.
- Exhale through your mouth, making a whooshing sound to a count of 8.
- Repeat until you feel calm in your body, mind, and nervous system.

Yoga also has a library of *asanas*, or poses, that can be very beneficial to help athletes with their recovery and their performance. As I mentioned earlier, I found yoga when I was so broken down I had no other options if I wanted to continue training and racing. Learning to slow down, take inventory of my body, and practice something without the intent to "win" was very counterintuitive at first. I laugh when I think of the competitive person who first showed up on the mat, frustrated at how inaccessible most of the poses were to me. It was a humbling process that helped me become the compassionate instructor I am now. Personally and professionally becoming a certified yoga instructor was hands down, the best post-college training I have done.

Finding an instructor that resonates with you and a practice that you enjoy will most certainly help you find your way more consistently to your yoga mat. There are many benefits of yoga for athletes, including: improved flexibility and mobility for more ease of movement, enhanced focus for the mental game, building resiliency, deepening your relationship with your body, improving functional strength and balance, using breath to enhance mental clarity, synchronizing movement, and calming the nervous system. It can also reveal imbalances in the body you may not be aware of, that if not addressed, could result in some form of injury. In all my years of teaching yoga to athletes, that reveal has been the biggest incentive to practice.

Stress can be a powerful motivator. It creates an environment for transformation. Just as carbon under immense pressure becomes a diamond, that pressure can reveal to us our greatness. Learning how to deal with, cope with, and see stress in a new way can help us achieve levels of performance—perhaps even levels that are unimaginable.

9. Deliberately rest and recover

Training + recovery from that training = improved performance

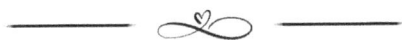

———— ∽◦◦ ————

Rest is not idleness, and to lie sometimes on the grass under trees on a summer's day, listening to the murmur of the water, or watching the clouds float across the sky, is by no means a waste of time.

—John Lubbock

———— ∽◦◦ ————

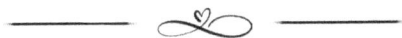

Rest and recovery are the partners of work, not the enemies. The same way you deliberately participate in your training, you must deliberately recover from it. The struggle and effort of training is familiar, and reward from it is expected. The quest for success and improved performance will work against you if you don't allow the adaptation that the stress pioneer Hans Selye tells us happens in recovery time. Stress without rest is unsustainable.

There is a simple formula to getting better in every aspect of any sport. There is hard work and then the necessary recovery from that hard work in order to get faster, stronger, leaner, jump higher, throw further, or whatever it is you are looking to do in your sport.

Recovery from training is eventually more important than the training itself. Repair and rebuilding of the damaged tissues from training can only occur during that time. Things like nutrition, sleep, even non-exercise stress reduction can help with recovery. If we all got to train, eat, sleep, rest, get massages, not have to work, raise families, and had no everyday life distractions, we would perform much better in competition and training. If you have ever had the luxury of being at a training camp, away from your everyday life and stressors, you may have found that you recovered much better in those ideal conditions when your non-exercise stressors were eliminated. Your neuromuscular system can only handle so much stress. When you take out non-exercise stress, there is more room for more exercise stress and more importantly, more room to recover from it.

So when most athletes want to experience better results, the first thing they do is to train harder. That is a good idea, until it isn't. The body can only take so much work until it has to recover and repair from that work. When you build a training program, there is a three hard/ one easy ratio that should be considered. Every four years, there is an Olympic Games. There is a three-year build and a one-year recovery. Every year, there should be nine months harder, three months easier. Every month, three weeks hard, one week recovery. Every week, three hard workouts, one easier.

> Take a moment to put that template on the past four years of your training plan, and I bet most of you have not adhered to that ratio. If you haven't crashed and burned yet, it may only be a matter of time.

The most challenging aspect that athletes may have is maintaining or improving their fitness and health while not accumulating fatigue to levels that will diminish their performance.

10. Take rest seriously

Overtraining can be compared to a delusional state and can be looked at as the equivalent of showing up to practice drunk. You may have thought your brain was working properly under the influence of alcohol when you made some very bad decisions, the same way you thought your body was performing fine under the influence of being overtrained and ended up injured or underperforming. We all know that the brain may think it is performing fine under the influence of alcohol, the same way the body thinks it is performing fine under the influence of being overtrained. Exercising with an addictive mind can destroy your body and your life.

Conscious athletes are at the forefront of the deliberate rest philosophy. They know that rest is a key to their success and take it very seriously, as seriously as their training.

Overtraining can be looked at another way: under-recovering. In my years of coaching, I have told many of my over-ly-stressed athletes that I would rather have them over-recovered at the starting line of a race than overtrained. For many, that is a tough concept to buy into and trust. The *more (work) is better* attitude, the familiar feeling of stress, the unconsciousness of ourselves and how we operate has led to looking for overtraining programs, with the supposed "reward" of fatigue and burnout as ways to, and guarantees of, optimal performance. Given that approach, there is no way for optimal performance to happen. The only way to perform your best is to manage the training stress with the recovery from it.

> Conscious athletes are at the forefront of the deliberate rest philosophy. They know that rest is a key to their success and take it very seriously, as seriously as their training.

Many of my athletes feel like they are being punished when I build an extra rest day into their week or taper them for a race more than they would like. "What do I do?" they ask. "I don't know what to do with myself if I'm not training." Learning to disconnect to recharge can be immensely rewarding. Taking a yoga class, getting a massage, meditating, and visualization are all strategies I encourage to help with their addiction to their sport. When you rest, it's an incubation period. It's like investing in your performance rather than paying a tax on it. We don't need to burn out to succeed. In fact, burning out will most definitely ensure you *won't* succeed.

The techniques for recovery can include everything from expensive, state-of-the-art equipment to simply getting more sleep. They can be short-term techniques such as a cool down at the end of the workout, foam rolling, post-exercise nutrition, and low-intensity exercise. Or they can be long-term techniques like periods of rest built into training from a weekly to an annual basis.

Restful sleep coupled with good nutrition and hydration help to restore homeostasis and full recovery. Humans are the only mammals that willingly delay sleep. When it comes to athletic performance, sleep plays a part in reaction times, motor function, motivation, focus, stress regulation, muscle recovery, sprint performance, muscle glycogen, glucose metabolism, memory and learning, injury risk, illness rates, and unwanted weight gain. The list could go on. More and more athletes are learning that sleep has a big impact on performance, wins, and losses. (Fatigue Science, 2015).

We now have the technology to monitor various physiological parameters in real time to measure and validate recovery and use the data collected to enhance the recovery process. For example, measuring resting heart rate (RHR), heart rate variability (HRV), and ventilation (breathing) patterns can provide valuable information on which nervous system is dominant, sympathetic (SNS), or parasympathetic (PNS). For recovery, we need to have PNS dominance where rest, repair, and recovery can happen.

Recovery strategies can vary from athlete to athlete, depending on things like the type of fatigue they are recovering from, other stressors in their life, and their training history. The more specific means of achieving recovery include active and nutritional recovery, cryo and hydrotherapy, massage, compression, and sleep. Athletes may use all of those strategies on a regular basis or different ones during different phases of their training.

11. Save your mental "energy"

When we work hard, we expect results. When we don't get the results we want, we work harder. If that doesn't work, we try to "make" it work. Like money invested, we hold high hopes for a profitable return. In understanding that there is a return not only on work, but also on recovery from that work, we can learn that not always pushing our bodies or stressing them beyond their limits, practicing patience, and detaching from outcome may produce the results we have been looking for. Work smarter, not harder.

Just as you have a bank account of money, you have a "body" account of energy. You have to save and spend and balance your account at the end of each month to make sure you have enough money or energy to pay your bills. If you are like most of us, the majority of your money goes to your home, car, kids, travel, or the things you love to do. The truth about our ATP (adenosine triphosphate, the energy molecule, or currency of energy in the body) is that 25 percent of it goes to your brain and 75 percent goes to your body. The brain uses energy daily at the rate of an athlete running a marathon. As you think, you use energy just like you do when you move your body.

Athletes use their bodies in a way that they feel is productive. They "spend" energy every day making their muscles work. The way we "spend" our thoughts is generally not that productive. Sometimes the investment of our thoughts is actually counterproductive when they create a reality that we have to overcome. It is very important to become aware of our thoughts because they are using energy. You have an energy budget, and if you write checks where you get no return for what you spend, you might as well give it away.

The 75 percent we spend on our physical bodies includes training. That amount is measurable for most athletes. Data, including how much power we can produce, what heart rates we train at, what pace we can hold, how long we can push, how far we can go, or how fast we can throw a ball, can all be measured and recorded along with any progress achieved. We understand the cost (calories or energy) and the benefit (improved fitness) and what we need to do to replenish the stores of ATP with nutrition, hydration, and rest. The 25 percent we spend on our mental processes are not so measurable or definable. Of course, after a long workout or training session, we not only replenish cells in our muscles, we also replenish our brain cells. Most of us have never considered the cost/benefit ratio to using our minds to enhance our performance or our lives.

We need to consider not just the energy needed for our brains to work, but also the reality we are creating with our thoughts. When you welcome in new awareness and make shifts in your consciousness, new ideas, thoughts, awareness and insight come into your mind and allow you to take new action. If you think of thoughts as snow, realize the snowman you are building is your reality. So let me leave you with that image of building the snowman you decide to create. I have many memories myself as a youngster growing up in Canada building snowmen that looked like they "should," and others that were more creative, fun, and whimsical. The creativity of stepping out of the familiar was exhilarating. I hope that this book also helps you find that same exhilaration of exploring other options on your road to a deeper awareness and higher consciousness of who you are and how sport helps you discover your full purpose and essence.

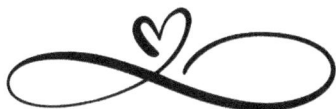

Epilogue:
The Hope for Humanity

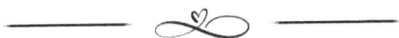

---

*It's in the convergence of spiritual people becoming
active, and active people becoming spiritual, that
the hope of humanity now rests.*

—Van Jones

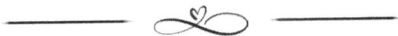

Sport is a way to develop a conscious awareness of who you are and where you are headed, why you are here and what your purpose is. You may be feeling a stirring from deep within yourself for change, to awaken to new possibilities and to grow. When you use the body as a platform to the soul, you have the ability to express your full potential. You understand that discomfort is necessary for learning to take place.

Most often, our way of being is simply memorized and unconsciously practiced—chronic familiar patterns. Create opportunities to step away from that familiarity into originality. See what new thoughts and new feelings can bring forth. Learning to become comfortable in the unknown is where growth and a new reality can find fertile soil to take root. It will take an open mind to question certainty, and when nothing is certain, anything is possible.

Moving inside of ourselves and digging into uncomfortable places is where we can break the habit of being the old, unconscious self and create the new, conscious, genuine self. When we have masked the truth of who we are, we must disassemble that mask to reveal that truth of our authentic nature.

Through sport, we have the privilege, if we so choose, to find our life purpose—not just our physical abilities. When you find out how far you can go, and you get there, there is no "there," and you understand limitations. Limitations are more often than not self-imposed and are opportunities to give us something to attempt to go beyond. If you believe you have infinite potential, who knows what you will be capable of in sport and in life.

When you see your performance more as a part of your journey than a definition of who you are, you have moved into the realm of consciousness and purpose. I am sure that most of you have put time, money, effort, perhaps your heart and soul into your sport. With that kind of endeavor, it is certainly possible that we are looking to satisfy the human longing for fulfillment, purpose, and to make sense out of our lives. Becoming conscious of what motivates you to that platform of purpose elevates you to a spiritual level of being.

Any kind of movement you may participate in through your sport will teach you more about yourself than you may even want to know. Sport allows you to gather pieces of understanding of yourself that you can only come to realize when you struggle. It helps you to see the self-image you have constructed in your reaction to feelings like frustration or joy. Do you practice gratitude or anger when you lose? Does winning ever bring you real joy? If you study yourself seriously enough, you will at some point come to realize that you are nearly always acting automatically, unconsciously. Of course there is value in that when you are learning physical skills. Practicing a movement pattern over and over will help you improve in your sport. But the thought, feeling, and belief patterns that are running on automatic over and over will eventually limit you if you are unaware of them, and they are what needs to change. The better we get to know ourselves, the less we fear change.

The Buddha tells us that as you think, you become; what you feel, you attract; and what you imagine, you create. Thoughts become words, words become actions, actions become habits, habits become character, and character becomes destiny.

If you haven't harnessed the power of your thoughts and feelings yet, your mind and your heart, you have not even begun to imagine what you can create and what your destiny can be. Along with the time you take to recover, take the time to investigate and be deliberate in what you think and feel. When you begin to question the thoughts you have and re-examine your reactions to every challenge, you are beginning to understand that you have the power to make the impossible possible.

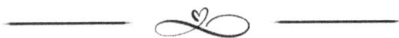

———— ♥∾ ————

If my mind can conceive it, and my heart can believe it, then I can achieve it.

—Mohammed Ali

———— ♥∾ ————

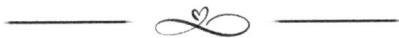

Thoughts become things. Learn to be deliberate in choosing them consciously rather than allowing them to unconsciously lead your life without your awareness of how off-course those thoughts may have taken you. Imagine if you spent even a fraction of the time training your mind as you do training your body. You would have the ability to powerfully move your mind and to still it. It would be a disciplined servant rather than an unruly dictator.

> *A Course in Miracles* tells us:
> *OUR THOUGHTS ARE NOT REAL(ITY)*
>
> Universal Principle tells us:
> *THOUGHTS BECOME THINGS*
>
> Therefore:
> *THOSE THINGS ARE NOT REAL(ITY)*
>
> *THE THOUGHTS WE HAVE...*
> *GO INTO OUR MINDS... AND BECOME THINGS*
> (Beliefs, life, reality, truth, habits, patterns, relationships...)
>
> *THE ONLY WAY TO CHANGE THOSE THINGS (REALITY)*
> *IS TO CHANGE THOSE THOUGHTS.*

Einstein can also be brought into the mix of this great message. He reminds us that we cannot solve our problems with the same thinking we used to create them. So, what needs to change? Yep. Our thoughts.

Remember John Locke's definition of consciousness: "...the perception of what passes through a man's mind." (Locke, 1690). Our mind is simply information the nervous system moves. That information sculpts our brain and creates our reality. When you become conscious of what information is moving through your mind, you can then choose to strengthen what serves you and weaken what doesn't. You get to decide what passes through and what reality you want to create. You know now that life isn't simply a projector and a movie screen. You get to shine the light of new awareness and consciousness through what film you deliberately decide to pass through your mind.

When you add in the power of your intuitive heart, you have a formula for creating possibilities you could never have even imagined before. The emotions of the heart also shape the patterns of the mind. Logic and emotion are powerful forces for good when you harness them. Choosing positive emotions to drive the direction of our thoughts is a skill that will create a whole new perception of how you can perform and live your life authentically and to your fullest potential.

—————— ❧⟳ ——————

I don't want to be at the mercy of my emotions.
I want to use them, to enjoy them, and
to dominate them.

—Oscar Wilde

—————— ❧⟳ ——————

Start to reside in the space between thoughts, the space between feelings, the space between each breath, the space between heartbeats. It is in that quiet space that peace and possibility exist.

You now know the steps. You have the tools. You have the means and the opportunity to make what was previously thought impossible, possible. Take baby steps, or cannonball into the pool—it's your choice as to how you want to wake up to your potential and the essence of who you really are as an athlete and a human being.

- Find new ways to do old things.
- Look through a new lens to evaluate difficult situations.
- Shift your perspective to find opportunities and solutions rather than obstacles and frustration. Do your best and then own it.
- No storytelling of how much better you "should" have done.
- Meet yourself where you are.
- Be dedicated to your practice and be flexible.
- Play and be curious, even if you feel masterful.
- Live more from intention than from habit.

Anything is possible when you decide to explore and be open. Change your thoughts, change your mind, change your feelings, change your reality.

You have powers you never dreamed of.
You can do things you never thought you could do.
There are no limitations in what you can do except
the limitations of your own mind.

—Darwin P. Kingsley

As you have navigated your way through this book, you have found what you need to do: explore and be open to a new way of thinking and feeling.

Once you set out on this journey of consciousness, you will find a whole new world of possibilities waiting for you. It's been there all along, waiting for you to bring it into your awareness and reality. Today, it is time for you to emerge as a conscious athlete and human being, to recognize yourself, your power, and your potential.

The beauty and power of expanding the consciousness of each athlete on the planet is most certainly welcomed and needed at this point in humanity. May you be inspired, believe anything is possible, and be more certain of your unique contribution to the world after reading this book.

Are you ready?

On your mark. Get set. Go!

Our deepest fear is not that we are inadequate.
Our deepest fear is that we are powerful
beyond measure.

—Marianne Williamson

A Reminder of Your Power...

I am here to remind you of your power of choice.
Of how your body is speaking to you. How it is
instructing you to find release. It offers a choice;
and in your choosing, it brings a response that
either brings more breath or stifles that breath.
It's time to remember your body's wisdom, dear one.
The intelligence that lives within you. The guide you
have been longing to meet.
It is here in your feeling heart.
Touch down into the pause... the wide open
and wise space. Find yourself here in the quiet.
Resting here in this peace, in this stillness, you will
feel your heart begin to awaken. To crack open.
To ignite into light.
You are built of body, mind, and spirit.
You are a perfect system of flawless structure
and force.
All is working to bring you into alignment and love,
into your highest state of being.
If you listen closely, you can feel your heart
expanding or contracting in each new moment and
movement.

—Sarah Blondin
https://www.sarahblondin.com/
A storyteller, author, and meditation guide
who unceasingly ruminates on the complexities
and nuances of life and the human heart.

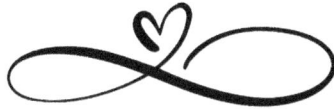

About the Author

Born and raised in Ottawa, Canada, Cindy found sport in her late teens as a competitive triathlete and canoe and flatwater kayak paddler. She attended The University of Ottawa, Queen's University and McArthur College, earning degrees in Exercise Physiology, Psychology, and Education. She has over 40 years of continued education and service to athletes as an educator, instructor, and coach, along with racing herself, from local fun events to World Championship level. Sport was a way for her to connect, to build friendship and community while living in different countries over those years. It was how she found meaning and realized her purpose in life.

Her education, experience, and insights have led her to develop a unique style and skillset to work with her athletes. A focus on finding purpose and growth; digging into motivation, mindset, strength, and mobility, along with a personal commitment to encouraging athletes to see beyond results, sets her apart from traditional coaching models.

She has worked with athletes from teens to over 70, including triathletes, rowers, runners, equestrians, paddlers, hockey players, swimmers, and stroke survivors.

Cindy walks her talk, and encourages her athletes to do the same. In guiding many athletes over the years to their athletic goals, she also encouraged them to see the bigger picture of their journey.

She sees herself as a midwife to the human spirit, helping people give birth to things from inside of them that they don't even know are there, through the vehicle of sport.

This book is her contribution to the evolution of human consciousness from its human to divine nature.

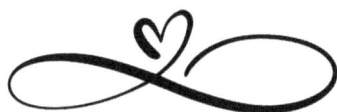

Call to Consciousness

Help the world and universe in the journey to expanding
consciousness.
The beauty and power of you is needed.
Answer the call.

www.cindydeugo.com
www.theconsciousathlete.com

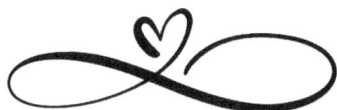

Book Club Questions for *The Power of a Conscious Athlete*

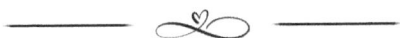

Simply put, there is nothing, nothing in the world that can take the place of one person intentionally listening or speaking to another.

—Jacob Needleman, Philosopher and Author

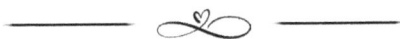

1. If you could ask the author one question after reading this book, what would it be?
2. Would you recommend this book to someone? Why or why not (with what caveats)?
3. Did you find the author's writing style easy to read? Why or why not? How long did it take you to get into the book?

4. What did you already know about this book's subject before reading it? What did you learn?
5. What aspect of the author's story did you most relate to?
6. What aspect of the book could you relate to the most?
7. What challenged you the most in this book? Do you believe anything is possible?
8. What feelings were evoked most powerfully for you from reading this book? Which part of the book and what emotion was felt?
9. Was the book thought-provoking? Did it change your opinion on anything? Did you learn something new you can apply to your own world?
10. What kind of reader would most enjoy this book?
11. Did you highlight or bookmark any passages from the book? Do you have a favorite quote or quotes? If so, share which and why?
12. Rate this book on a scale of 1 to 10, with 10 being the highest. Why did you give the book the rating you did? Did any part of this book club discussion change your rating from what it would have been directly after finishing the book?
13. Compare this book to others you have read covering similar topics. How are they the same? How are they different?

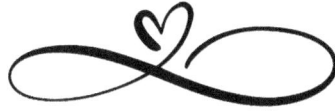

References

Allen, James. *As a Man Thinketh.* Mount Vernon, N.Y.: Peter Pauper Press, 1951.

Bauer, Brent, MD, Mayo Clinic, 2022, How Meditation Changes the Brain. https://www.thorne.com/take-5-daily/article/how-meditation-changes-the-brain.

Bone, Muscle, and Joint Team. 2022. "How Do Your Bones Change over Time?" Health Essentials from Cleveland Clinic. Health Essentials from Cleveland Clinic. April 4, 2022. https://health.clevelandclinic.org/how-do-your-bones-change-over-time.

"Breathing." 2014. The Lung Association. August 20, 2014. https://www.lung.ca/lung-health/lung-info/breathing.

Broadwell, Martin, 1969, Teaching for Learning (XVI.). *Gospel Guardian* vol. 20, no. 41.

Byrne, John, 2020. "Learning and Memory (Section 4, Chapter 7) Neuroscience Online: An Electronic Textbook for the Neurosciences | Department of Neurobiology and Anatomy – the University of Texas Medical School at Houston." n.d. Nba.uth.tmc.edu. https://nba.uth.tmc.edu/neuroscience/m/s4/chapter07.html.

Covey, Stephen, Robert Merrill and Rebecca Merrill. *First Things First, To Live, To Love, To Learn, To Leave a Legacy.* NY: Free Press, 1996

Ehrmann, J, and G Jordan. *Inside Out Coaching - How Sport Can Transform Lives,* Simon and Schuster, 2011

Emerald, David. *The Power of TED : The Empowerment Dynamic.* Bainbridge Island, Wa: Polaris Publishing, 2016

Fallah, M., Moghadas Tabrizi, Y., Gharayagh Zandi, H. The Effects of Neurofeedback training on Attention and performance in free throw skill. *Neuropsychology*, 2018; 4(13): 97–108.

Fischetti, Mark, and Jen Christiansen. "Our Bodies Replace Billions of Cells Every Day." *Scientific American*, April 2021. https://doi.org/10.1038/scientificamerican0421-76.

Foundation For Inner Peace. *A Course in Miracles: Combined Volume.* New York: Viking, 1996.

Glattfelder, J.B. (2019). The Consciousness of Reality. In: Information—Consciousness—Reality. The Frontiers Collection. Springer, Cham. https://doi.org/10.1007/978-3-030-03633-1_14

Gallowey, Timothy. *The Inner Game of Tennis: The Classic Guide to the Mental Side of Peak Performance.* Random House Trade Paperbacks, 1997.

Goleman, Daniel, and Richard J Davidson. *Altered Traits : Science Reveals How Meditation Changes Your Mind, Brain, and Body.* NY: Avery, An Imprint Of Penguin Random House LLC, 2017.

Gollwitzer, P. M. (1999). Implementation intentions: Strong effects of simple plans. *American Psychologist, 54*(7), 493–503. https://doi.org/10.1037/0003-066X.54.7.493.

Hadfield, Chris. *An Astronaut's Guide to Life on Earth.* Little, Brown, 2013.

Hallbom, Kris, and Tim Hallbom. "Exploring the Neuroscience and Magic Behind Setting Your Intent – And Creating an Optimal Future for Yourself." NLP Institute of California. April 10, 2012, https://nlpca.com/creating-an-optimal-future-for-yourself/

Hammond. D. Corydon (2011) What is Neurofeedback: An Update, Journal of Neurotherapy: Investigations in Neuromodulation, Neurofeedback and Applied Neuroscience, 15:4, 305–336, DOI: 10.1080/10874208.2011.62.

Harvard Health Publishing, Harvard Medical School, 2020. https://www.health.harvard.edu/staying-healthy/ understanding-the-stress-response.

Hawkins, David MD Ph.D (2013) Power vs Force – The Hidden Determinants of Human Behavior, Hay House.

Hawkins, David R. *Power vs. Force : The Hidden Determinants of Human Behavior, Author's Official Revised Edition.* Carlsbad: Hay House Publishing, 2013.

Hughes, Clara. *Open Heart, Open Mind.* Canada: Simon and Schuster, 2017.

Jensen, Peter.. *Ignite the Third Factor.* Thomas Allen Publishers, 2011.

Klein, Nadav, and Ed O'Brien. 2017. "The Power and Limits of Personal Change: When a Bad Past Does (and Does Not) Inspire in the Present." *Journal of Personality and Social Psychology* 113 (2): 210–29. https://doi.org/10.1037/pspa0000088.

Koo, Patrick. "The CO2 Tolerance Test and Why You Should Be Working On Your Lungs." Cruxfit. September 30, 2019. https://www.cruxfit.com/the-co2-tolerance-test-and-why-you-should-be-working-on-your-lungs.

Koster, Maranke I. 2009. "Making an Epidermis." *Annals of the New York Academy of Sciences* 1170 (July): 7–10. https://doi. org/10.1111/j.1749-6632.2009.04363.x.

Lally, Phillippa & Jaarsveld, Cornelia & Potts, Henry & Wardle, Jane. 2010. How are habits formed: Modeling habit formation in the real world. European Journal of Social Psychology. 40. 10.1002/ejsp.674.

Lipton, Bruce H. *The Biology of Belief : Unleashing the Power of Consciousness, Matter & Miracles.* Carlsbad, Calif.: Hay House, 2008.

Locke, John. *An Essay Concerning Human Understanding.* WLC, 2009.

Luft, Joseph, *Of Human Interaction.* Palo Alto, Calif., National Press Books, 1969.

McCraty, Rollin, Ph.D, 2015, Science of the Heart - Exploring the Role of the Heart in Human Performance, Vol 2, HeartMath™ Institute.

McCraty, Rollin. (2003). The Energetic Heart: Biolectromagnetic Interactions Within and Between People. The Neuropsychotherapist. 6. 22–43. 10.12744/tnpt(6)022-043.

Nerurkar, Aditi, Asaf Bitton, Roger B. Davis, Russell S. Phillips, and Gloria Yeh. 2013. "When Physicians Counsel about Stress: Results of a National Study." *JAMA Internal Medicine* 173 (1): 76. https://doi.org/10.1001/2013.jamainternmed.480.

Northern Illinois University Center for Innovative Teaching and Learning. 2020. Howard Gardner's theory of multiple intelligences. In *Instructional guide for university faculty and teaching assistants.* Retrieved from https://www.niu.edu/citl/resources/guides/instructional-guide.

Nummenmaa, L., E. Glerean, R. Hari, and J. K. Hietanen. 2013. "Bodily Maps of Emotions." *Proceedings of the National Academy of Sciences* 111 (2): 646–51. https://doi.org/10.1073/pnas.1321664111.

Oettinger, Gabrielle. *Rethinking Positive Thinking: Inside the New Science of Motivation, Current.* NY: Penguin Random House, 2015

Orlick, Terry, and John Partington. 1988. "Mental Links to Excellence." *The Sport Psychologist* 2 (2): 105–30. https://doi.org/10.1123/tsp.2.2.105.

Chödrön, Pema, *Start Where You Are: A Guide to Compassionate Living.* Boston, Shambhala, 1994.

Peters, Steve. *The Chimp Paradox: The Mind Management Program to Help You Achieve Success, Confidence, and Happiness.* New York: Penguin, a member of Penguin Group Inc, 2013.

Queensland Brain Institute at the University of Queensland, Brain-Facts-QBI-poster-QBI-UQ.pdf.

Roche, Joyce. *The Empress Has No Clothes: Conquering Self Doubt to Embrace Success*. San Francisco, CA: Berrett-Koehler Publishers, Inc., 2013.

Russell, Peter, The Reality of Consciousness, https://www.peterrussell.com/SCG/realityconsc.php.

Santarnecchi, Emiliano, Sicilia D'Arista, Eutizio Egiziano, Concetta Gardi, Roberta Petrosino, Giampaolo Vatti, Mario Reda, and Alessandro Rossi. "Interaction between neuroanatomical and psychological changes after mindfulness-based training." *PloS one* 9, no. 10 (2014): e108359.

Review of *The Word "Power" Is Rooted in the Old French Pouvoir: To Be Able, and Latin Potus: Powerful (Etymology Dictionary 2021)*. n.d. In *Etymology Dictionary*.

Review of *Force on the Other Hand Is Rooted in Old French Forcer: Conquer by Violence, Exert Force upon (Etymology Dictionary 2021)*. n.d. In *Etymology Dictionary*.

Science, Fatigue. 2015. "5 Areas Sleep Has the Greatest Impact on Athletic Performance." Fatigue Science. September 24, 2015. https://fatiguescience.com/blog/5-ways-sleep-impacts-peak-athletic-performance.

Selye, Hans. 1936. "A Syndrome Produced by Diverse Nocuous Agents." *Nature* 138 (3479): 32–32. https://doi.org/10.1038/138032a0.

Singer, Michael A. *The untethered soul the journey beyond yourself*. Oakland, CA: New Harbinger Publications, 2007.

Sullivan, John, and Chris Parker. *The Brain Always Wins*. Urbane Publications, 2016

Tang, Rongxiang, Karl J. Friston, and Yi-Yuan Tang. 2020. "Brief Mindfulness Meditation Induces Gray Matter Changes in a Brain Hub." Edited by Wei-Lin Liu. *Neural Plasticity*, 2020 (November): 1–8. https://doi.org/10.1155/2020/8830005.

Texas Heart Institute. 2018. "Heart Information Center: Heart Anatomy | Texas Heart Institute." Texas Heart Institute. 2018. https://www.texasheart.org/heart-health/heart-information-center/topics/heart-anatomy.

Tseng, J., Poppenk, J. Brain meta-state transitions demarcate thoughts across task contexts

exposing the mental noise of trait neuroticism. *Nat Commun* 11, 3480, 2020.

Tyng CM, Amin HU, Saad MNM, Malik AS. The Influences of Emotion on Learning and Memory. Front Psychol. 2017 Aug 24; 8:1454. doi: 10.3389/fpsyg.2017.01454. PMID: 28883804; PMCID: PMC5573739.

Warren, Rick. *The Purpose-Driven Life : What on Earth Am I Here for?* Grand Rapids, Mich.: Zondervan, 2002.

"What Is Meditation? – 2016 North American Kagyu Monlam." n.d. Kagyumonlamny.org. Accessed November 21, 2022. https://kagyumonlamny.org/what-is-meditation.

Yeo SS, Chang PH, Jang SH. The ascending reticular activating system from pontine reticular formation to the thalamus in the human brain. Front Hum Neurosci. 2013 Jul 25;7:416. doi: 10.3389/fnhum.2013.00416. PMID: 23898258; PMCID: PMC3722571.

"Definition of MEDITATE." n.d. Www.merriam-Webster.com. https://www.merriam-webster.com/dictionary/meditate.

The B Corp Movement

Dear reader,

Thank you for reading this book and joining the Publish Your Purpose community! You are joining a special group of people who aim to make the world a better place.

What's Publish Your Purpose About?

Our mission is to elevate the voices often excluded from traditional publishing. We intentionally seek out authors and storytellers with diverse backgrounds, life experiences, and unique perspectives to publish books that will make an impact in the world.

Certified

Beyond our books, we are focused on tangible, action-based change. As a woman- and LGBTQ+-owned company, we are committed to reducing inequality, lowering levels of poverty, creating a healthier environment, building stronger communities, and creating high-quality jobs with dignity and purpose.

Corporation

As a Certified B Corporation, we use business as a force for good. We join a community of mission-driven companies building a more equitable, inclusive, and sustainable global economy. B Corporations must meet high standards of transparency, social and environmental performance, and accountability as determined by the nonprofit B Lab. The certification process is rigorous and ongoing (with a recertification requirement every three years).

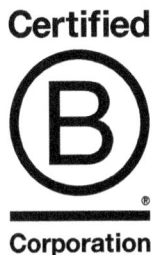

How Do We Do This?

We intentionally partner with socially and economically disadvantaged businesses that meet our sustainability goals. We embrace and encourage our authors and employee's differences in race, age, color, disability, ethnicity, family or marital status, gender identity or expression, language, national origin, physical and mental ability, political affiliation, religion, sexual orientation, socio-economic status, veteran status, and other characteristics that make them unique.

Community is at the heart of everything we do—from our writing and publishing programs to contributing to social enterprise nonprofits like reSET (https://www.resetco.org/) and our work in founding B Local Connecticut.

We are endlessly grateful to our authors, readers, and local community for being the driving force behind the equitable and sustainable world we are building together.

To connect with us online, or publish with us,
visit us at www.publishyourpurpose.com.

Elevating Your Voice,

Jenn T Grace

Jenn T. Grace
Founder, Publish Your Purpose